The JCAHO Alternative

The JCAHO Alternative

Steve Wilkinson, Michael Carlisle, and Wanda Morgan

2006

The JCAHO Alternative

Table of Contents

Table of Contents

Preface

The purpose of this book is to provide information and insight into alternative choices for healthcare-facility accreditation. Healthcare management textbooks and articles on accrediting alternatives tend to be rather limited. Most health executives think primarily of the Joint Commission on Accreditation of Healthcare Organizations (JCAHO) when they are questioned about hospital accreditation, or the National Committee for Quality Assurance (NCQA) as an obvious choice for managed care facilities. When executives are questioned about Conditions of Participation (CoP) for federal reimbursement under the Medicare program or federal/state reimbursement under the state Medicaid program, the above two organizations would also be at the top of their lists. But when they are informed that CoP for Medicare and Medicaid can be met through accreditation from the Healthcare Facilities Accreditation Program (HFAP), they generally respond that they have never heard of it or that they understand that HFAP only accredits osteopathic facilities.

There are over 6,500 general and specialty hospitals in the United States. JCAHO, an independent nonprofit organization, conducts quality assessment and accreditation for 80 percent of all of them and for over 6,000 other healthcare facilities such as mental health organizations, long-term-care facilities, and outpatient surgery centers.

There is no doubt that even with the concerns expressed over the years by healthcare action groups, lobbyists, and Capitol Hill, JCAHO has and continues to be a significant healthcare accrediting organization. But for those healthcare organizations and executives who question whether there are alternatives, the answer is an emphatic yes!

The contents of this book will be an unbiased view of HFAP as an accrediting organization and peer to JCAHO. As a healthcare facility reviewer organization, HFAP has been in existence longer than JCAHO and it has the same deeming credentials from the Centers for Medicare and Medicaid Services (CMS); however, its profile has been low for all those years, and it does not enjoy the brand recognition of the larger organization.

Chapter one provides an introduction to the importance of Medicare reimbursement and its impact on the healthcare industry followed by a brief summary of the evolution of U.S. medicine and details of the changes that medical care has had on the hospital movement. This chapter also traces the history of medical education and an introduction to quality and standardization.

Measuring quality in any field is complicated, but nowhere is it more so than in medicine. Chapter two provides some history of quality and its relationship to healthcare institutions. Making certain that patient care "does no harm" is more important than in any other industry because human lives are at stake. The desire for improved quality in healthcare has driven the impulse to accredit, to certify, and to credential. It is out of these concerns that accreditation associations were born. An understanding of the developments that led to them is useful to administrators in making decisions for their own institutions.

Chapter three details the history of The Healthcare Facilities Accreditation Program (HFAP) and explains its survey process. This accrediting program of the American Osteopathic Association has had a low profile in the history of Medicare even though it was granted deeming authority from the outset of the enactment of Title XVIII of the Social Security Act and slightly after JCAHO. However, in recent years allopathic hospitals have begun not only to discover it, but also to see it as either an attractive add-on for programs that may not be appropriate for accreditation through JCAHO or as an alternative to JCAHO for facility accreditation. HFAP is considered by many to conduct surveys that are more effective in achieving the goal of continuous quality, cost-effectiveness, and user-friendliness.

JCAHO has long been considered the gold standard for accreditation of healthcare facilities in this country, and has also been recruited in other countries to improve the quality of their own healthcare institutions. Its tumultuous history is detailed in chapter four, and along with the dynamic nature of our healthcare system, the many changes and iterations of JCAHO are expressed as well. It has gone from the careful measurer and evaluator of process to collaborator in continuous quality improvement with a focus on outcomes. Medicare mandated that all surveys be unannounced beginning January 1, 2006, so both HFAP and JCAHO have made changes in their survey approaches. These changes are explained in Chapters 3 and 4.

Chapter five announces a potential newcomer to healthcare accreditation. TÜV, an American quality-management company with ties to the quality movement in Europe, has been providing consulting services to many hospitals in this country for several years and has applied to Medicare for deeming authority. This chapter briefly identifies TÜV, where it came from, and what it offers.

Chapter six compares accreditation options for hospitals and other healthcare facilities in terms of influence on marketing to a community, attracting medical staff members, and cost, to name a few key factors. Though it is an unscientific comparison, it does provide key elements that should be taken into account when considering an initial or re-accreditation option.

Chapter seven draws conclusions based on our assessment of the materials presented throughout the previous chapters.

It is the intention of this book to serve as useful information for key administrators and managers for decision making when it comes to accreditation needs, or at the very least, to provoke other questions and concerns that can be addressed in further detail. It is noted that the expressed and implied views of this book are solely those of its authors and not necessarily those of the accrediting agencies discussed. We acknowledge those who have contributed to the content to this book. For further information please contact Mr. Stephen Wilkinson at swilkinson@hcqagroup.com or Mr. Michael A. Carlisle at mcarlisle@hcqagroup.com.

Chapter 1
Development, Growth, and Standardization of the U.S. Hospital

Hospitals and Traditional Medicare Reimbursement

There was a time when the hospitalization of patients with burdening lengths of stay was the norm. Advances in medical technology and procedures coupled with improved drug therapies have helped reduce the amount of time patients spend in hospitals. The promotion of healthier lifestyles may also have some influence on inpatient lengths of stay. Tighter controls on health-insurance reimbursements may also be a factor. Costly hospital stays tend to be reserved for only the sickest of the sick. In many instances, these are patients who are supported by Medicare Part A (hospital services) and Part B (medical insurance). To put this in some perspective, the U.S. Agency for Healthcare Research and Quality reported that in 2003 our nation's hospitals billed insurers and consumers nearly $754 billion, of which Medicare's bill for inpatient care amounted to $327 billion or roughly 43 percent of the total charges.[1] These numbers make the traditional

Medicare fee for service (FFS) program one of the most important and sometimes the most complex aspect of fiscal management for Medicare-accepting healthcare facilities and the administrators that manage them.

Today's chief administrator must constantly weigh many factors that influence decisions regarding expenditures and investments. For example, if the radiology department does not have state-of-the-art equipment, physicians will send their patients to a hospital that does. If the oncology department is not practicing the most current procedures, primary care physicians will cease to refer their patients. But often the most important factor in the mix is reimbursements. With many companies no longer providing top-of-the-line health insurance for employees and with high demands to provide charity care for patients with little or no health insurance, keeping the institution in the black becomes increasingly complicated. With the potential for a high census of elderly patients, a hospital cannot survive without reimbursement from Medicare for services provided to the elderly and disabled patients; so first and foremost, the administrator must do whatever is necessary to secure and maintain that reimbursement.

So how does a hospital administrator manage this part of the business? First of all, the hospital must meet the CMS's qualification standards for reimbursement as defined by the Medicare Conditions of Participation (CoP). There are three major options for demonstrating compliance: a State Survey conducted on behalf of CMS; accreditation by the Joint Commission on Accreditation of Healthcare Organizations (JCAHO); or accreditation by the Healthcare Facilities Accreditation Program (HFAP), an arm of the American Osteopathic Association. These two accrediting associations have been given "deeming" authority by CMS to conduct hospital accrediting surveys on its behalf. CMS accepts accreditation by these two associations as evidence that the healthcare institution is in compliance with the CoP. But how did we get to the point of hospitals and other healthcare facilities subjecting themselves to voluntary accreditation standards in order to receive federal reimbursements?

The Development of the American Hospital

Scientific Progress

It was a Frenchman named Louis Pasteur who was partially responsible for the advancement in medicine that brought about the revolution in the hospitals in this country in the 19th century. Strangely enough, this remarkable scientist's development of the "germ theory of disease" began with a study of wine. A distiller named Bigo asked for Pasteur's help in solving the problem of contaminants, and Pasteur found the answer. He identified specific microorganisms that could be cultivated—new knowledge at that time and the basis for the field of microbiology. He moved on from there to demonstrate that transmittable infectious agents that could be controlled by sterilization caused many of the most dangerous diseases. Armed with this new knowledge about infection, the most common cause of mortalities in surgery patients, American physicians began to improve surgery in this country.

Added to Pasteur's breakthrough were discoveries about anatomy and physiology that changed diagnosis from mostly educated guesses and conjecture to fact-based evaluations. Soon to follow was the discovery of anesthesia, which made it possible for a surgeon to take more time in performing an operation to make certain he was thorough and complete, and the revolution was launched. From the beginning of the 19th Century when surgery was a very primitive art to the end of that century when surgical professionals were armed with a new arsenal of weapons, survival rates following surgeries soared. Once the diseases were under control and better understood, pre- and post-operative care led to a greater need for hospital beds and personnel. By 1900, surgeries accounted for a large percentage of hospitalizations.

Technology

These new understandings and successes led to more interest in research and development, and invention and experimentation in new technologies grew. Laboratories became a vital part of the services demanded by the doctors, and hospitals began to add them. X-ray was first used to diagnose illness in 1896. In 1901, blood types were discovered, and in 1903 the electrocardiogram was used for the first time. By 1929, the electroencephalogram was being used. By this time, hospitals as asylums for the poor and indigent had been replaced by modern treatment centers where everyone came to be healed, not just the poor and indigent.

The physician of the past was also being replaced by a group of doctors since all of this equipment couldn't be carried around in a bag. Instead of a sole practitioner providing for patients on his own, a network of specialists was in place to provide the range of skills and knowledge required in this new environment. And it was in the hospital where it all came together.

Nursing

Since hospitals were charitable institutions, care was provided by Catholic nuns or Protestant deaconesses whose dedication could not be disputed, but whose training for their jobs was sparse. Many of the welfare institutions were staffed by unskilled and poorly paid workers, very often people who could not find and hold jobs elsewhere.

It was another foreigner, this time a British woman, who brought about the next major change in hospital care in the United States as well as around the world. Florence Nightingale was born in Italy in 1820 but grew up in Hampshire, England.

Untypical for her time, she was well educated, particularly in mathematics. Her use of statistical analysis to plot mortality rates and to dramatize unsanitary conditions brought about the next major change in American hospitals. She wrote about her experiences in the Crimean War and the efforts she and the other nurses had made to use cleanliness, sanitation, and other means to save lives. In 1860, she founded the Nightingale School for Nursing in England. The message did not go unheard in America.

Hospital training for nurses was introduced in America at the time of the Civil War. After the war ended, schools of nursing opened at Bellevue Hospital, New Haven Hospital, and Massachusetts General. Administrators were not enthusiastic at first but soon came to see how much difference the trained nurses made in the welfare of patients. By 1898, 400 schools were in operation in this country and 10,000 graduates were serving in hospitals.

The improvement in nursing care impacted the hospital business in several ways. For one, hospitals began to be seen not as asylums for the poor and indigent but as the best possible place for all sick people to receive care regardless of class. Mortality and morbidity rates went down because of the improvements in sanitation and diet, not to mention the replacing of the haphazard care of the past with formal routines. This transformation in nursing generated greater confidence in the hospitals.

Medical Education

In the 19ᵗʰ Century, medical education was obtained in three ways: a sort of apprenticeship with a local physician; a proprietary school with lectures by the doctor-owners; or a program in a university that included classes and clinical practice in a university-related hospital. The types of medicine taught were diverse and included such divisions as scientific, osteopathic, homeopathic, etc. Wealthier students would sometimes go to a university in Europe for more training. The result of this situation was a hodgepodge of approaches to care. The American Medical Association (AMA) sought to standardize medical education and appealed to the Carnegie Foundation for the Advancement of Teaching to conduct such a study.

Abraham Flexner, not a physician but an educator, was chosen to conduct the study, which resulted in a report entitled "Medical Education in the United States and Canada," popularly titled the Flexner Report, which brought about dramatic changes not only in the education of physicians but in the hospitals where they would study and practice. Flexner took three years to study and write his report and visited 155 medical schools, examining entrance requirements, size and training of the faculty, endowment and tuition, laboratories, and access to a teaching hospital. He reported that very few American medical schools had the resources to provide what was needed. Moreover, he found that the range between the best and the worst was vast. He recommended that properly supported institutions replace commercial schools.

The hospital business underwent yet another transformation as the result of the Flexner report. The role of the hospital was no longer limited to patient care but grew to include education and research. As specialties proliferated, so did the demands for more and more space and equipment. Residencies and internships increased dramatically during the 1920s and 1930s. The changes brought about by the Flexner Report included improved medical care for patients, particularly those with illnesses that were difficult to diagnose and treat.

Quality Concerns and Movement towards Standardization and Accreditation

In the early years of the 20th century, healthcare in hospitals was very primitive. Patients were primarily indigents and the conditions were often similar to those in a cheap hotel. Few patients were examined at the time of admission, no history was taken, no diagnosis made, and the notion of follow-up played no part in the treatment provided. For that reason, medical records were irrelevant. Also, physician competence was never questioned; and since medical staffs were not organized, there was no mechanism for managing the care being provided. In addition, few hospitals had clinical laboratories or radiology services or any other means of conducting studies either pre- or post-operative.

This is not to say that the medical professionals of that time were not concerned about the conditions in hospitals. The surgeons, in particular, were working to improve the situation and were optimistic that a hospital system could be developed that would provide orderly care for patients with acute illness and would be effective in restoring health for most of them. Progress was being made. The introduction of antiseptic surgery, for instance, brought about dramatic improvements in outcomes. At the same time, many of the surgeons were convinced that some measure of standardization had to be achieved if hospitals were to carry out their missions of rendering the best possible care and treatment for their patients. In 1917, a three-day conference was held in Chicago that brought together three hundred American College of Surgeons (ACS) fellows and sixty hospital superintendents for this express purpose. Following that meeting, a committee made up of 21 members went to work on a hospital evaluation questionnaire and a minimum standard.

It's not surprising that it was the surgeons who got the ball rolling on accreditation. In the early years of the 20th century, medicine had few answers for most of the illnesses that were fatal or disabling. For example, although high blood pressure was recognized as a killer, there was no treatment available to control it. Most patients who ended up in hospitals were there for surgical procedures of one kind or another.

Two surgeons, Dr. Ernest Codman of Boston and Dr. Edward Martin of Philadelphia were in England to meet with the Royal College of Surgeons about founding an ACS in the summer of 1910. Dr. Codman had a theory that he called "End Result System of Hospital Organization," which was simply that hospitals should follow patients long enough to be sure the treatment was successful and to answer the question, "if not, why not?" The two surgeons felt that creating the College of Surgeons would be a good way to introduce this idea into hospitals and to achieve some standardization.

From this beginning, the movement toward the eventual accrediting of hospitals emerged. The ACS was founded in 1913 with the need for hospital standards its most pressing concern. This early work by the surgeons led to a quickly expanding effort to develop an accrediting system to improve the quality of hospitals. In 1951, the American College of Physicians (ACP), the American Hospital Association (AHA), the AMA, and the Canadian Medical Association joined with the ACS to form the Joint Commission on Accreditation of Hospitals (JCAH), now the Joint Commission on Accreditation of Healthcare Organizations (JCAHO). Eventually, Canada split off to form its own system, but JCAHO continued to develop and expand.

In 1943, the American Osteopathic Association (AOA) began to develop its own accrediting program, which it implemented in 1945 as the AOA Accreditation Program, now known as the Healthcare Facilities Accreditation Program (HFAP). Under HFAP, hospitals were surveyed each year to assure that osteopathic students who were receiving their training through rotating internships and residencies were in institutions that provided a high quality of patient care. When Medicare was introduced in 1965, HFAP was granted deeming authority to survey hospitals for compliance with the Medicare CoP followed by JCAHO. It should also be noted that HFAP is a recognized alternative to accreditation by CMS or JCAHO.

The drive for medical excellence in this country has culminated in what has sometimes been called the finest medical system in the world. There were heroes along the way, not the least of which were the presidents who staked their political careers on their support of a system that would meet the healthcare needs of those who needed it most and could afford it least—the elderly and the poor. Today, gall bladder removal (cholecystectomy), which in the past called for several days in a hospital room for recovery, is a same-day outpatient procedure. Hearts are repaired and productive years extended. Outcomes in the case of infectious disease epidemics such as the influenza that killed millions in 1918 are much more optimistic thanks to the very complex system of antibiotics administered by highly skilled 21st-century medical practitioners.

The management of the institutions that provide healthcare has become unbelievably complex. At the same time, the efforts to assure quality of care through accreditation of hospitals that was initiated by Dr. Codman and Dr. Martin after their trip to England in 1910 has evolved and continues to promote excellence in the nation's healthcare institutions.

Chapter 2
Quality Standards Overview and its Significance to Medicare Participation

Standard setting is complicated in any human endeavor; in medicine, where change and progress are the norm, it is perhaps the most difficult of all. The Christian reformers of the 16th Century declared that religion should be reformed but always reforming, and so it is with medicine. Medical professionals in any area—be they generalists or specialists—must devote much of their professional time to keeping up with the latest discoveries, challenges, and developments.

Industrialization brought about an unprecedented explosion of knowledge about illnesses at the end of the 19th Century. Scientists were becoming aware of the role that infection played in deadly diseases such as anthrax, gonorrhea, malaria, pneumonia, typhoid fever, tetanus, influenza, etc. The sudden burst of knowledge about the causes of many of the hitherto mysterious and dreaded afflictions spawned optimism that they might be prevented and even successfully treated. Advances in anesthesia and antisepsis were also being made at an accelerated rate. At the same time, the development of diagnostic tools such as x-rays was transforming the work of surgeons.

A movement to improve medical care was gathering steam in many sectors. It's not surprising, then, that Drs. Codman and Martin in 1910 determined that North America needed a college of surgeons. The AMA, founded in 1847, was already campaigning to raise standards in medical education, medical ethics, and state licensing. Abraham Flexner of the Carnegie Foundation published a report on medical education in 1910 recommending that schools work directly with hospitals in the training of surgeons since at that time medical college graduates often had no experience at all in seeing or caring for patients.

These advances spawned the creation of many new hospitals during this period not only by philanthropic groups such as churches and women's groups but also by cities and counties, even states. Physicians, who had the greatest stake in how the facilities were managed, staffed, and equipped, were also building their own hospitals

At the same time that Codman was promoting his End Result theories, many other industries were also becoming interested in efficiency and standardization. Engineering, for example, promoted observation, measurement, precision, perfectibility, and results. The National Bureau of Standards, established by the U.S. Department of Commerce in 1901, emerged from this movement. Codman and Martin were members of a new generation of scientifically-oriented doctors who intended to make the discoveries and knowledge emerging from the other professional fields a part of the new medicine of the new century.

Martin established the journal *Surgery, Gynecology & Obstetrics* in 1905 as the first foray into the dissemination of a dogma of specialist medicine. The first Clinical Congress of Surgeons in Chicago in 1910 was so successful that attendance had to be limited at subsequent ones in 1911 in Philadelphia and New York in 1912. Almost immediately, the question arose as to whether it was more important to bring the skills of all doctors up to a minimally acceptable standard or to create a small, recognizable group of stars. Out of all of this came the move to require surgical certification beyond the medical degree and to create special licensure for surgeons.

The AMA was lukewarm to these changes because most of its members were general practitioners who were already licensed to perform surgery. They were concerned that their own professional images might suffer and were fearful of losing the income they derived from performing surgical procedures. Ultimately, while the AMA continued to work on eliminating the inferior medical schools, it held the line on credentialing. However, the efforts of the AMA to improve medical education did result in a decrease in the number of medical schools from 155 in 1909 to 76 in 1930.

In 1912, the New York Clinical Congress of Surgeons decreed that a system for standardizing hospital equipment and hospital work should be developed; and when the ACS was formed in 1912, hospital standardization was its stated purpose.

In 1914, John G. Bowman, Ph.D., succeeded Dr. Codman as chairman of the Hospital Standardization Committee of the ACS and secured a $30,000 grant from Carnegie Foundation to underwrite the beginnings of a hospital standardization program. A meeting between three hundred ACS fellows and sixty leading hospital superintendents in 1917 addressed standardization priorities and established the principle that hospital conditions should be assessed by knowledgeable professionals who should try to achieve consensus on standards that would have the greatest effect on improving patient care. Following the meeting, a 21-member committee set out to formulate a minimum standard by sending a questionnaire to 2,700 hospitals in the United States and Canada.

In the first six months of 1919, Bowman, his staff, and members of state standardization committees held 20 conferences to explain the objectives of the ACS. To say that the efforts of Bowman and his colleagues were not well received is an understatement; hospitals did not want anyone telling them how they should be running their businesses. Even so, in October of that year, Bowman reported the dismal results of the field trials run by standardization committee personnel. Of the 692 hospitals of 100 beds or more that had been examined, only 89 met the minimum standards that the ACS had determined should be a baseline. Only 264 held regular staff meetings and only 301 kept case records. The list was burned in the furnace of the Waldorf-Astoria Hotel to prevent word from getting out about which hospitals were performing at acceptable standards and which were not.

However, the aggregate numbers were published and in the long run achieved the advancement of standardization. Bowman's committee quickly drafted and published the minimum standard, which had only five points:

- Physicians and surgeons with hospital privileges should be organized as a definite group of staff.
- Staff membership should be restricted to graduates of medical schools in good standing and to those licensed, competent, and worthy in character and in matters of professional ethics.
- The staff should initiate and, with the approval of the hospital's governing board, adopt rules, regulations, and policies governing the professional work of the hospital, including requirements that staff meetings be held at least monthly and that the staff review and analyze at regular intervals the clinical experience of departments.
- Accurate and complete case records should be written for all patients, filed in the hospital, and made easily accessible.
- Diagnostic and therapeutic facilities including a clinical laboratory and an x-ray department under competent supervision should be available for the study, diagnosis, and treatment of patients.[2]

In 1920, seven doctors, instructed to collect facts but also to be constructive and helpful, were in the field doing evaluations. There was still some dispute about whether the purpose was to evaluate or to teach, but by January, the ACS was ready to publish the results. In 1920, 29 percent of the hospitals met the standard; in 1921, 76 percent; and in 1922, 83 percent.

Thus the groundwork was laid for the development of the enormously complicated system of standardization that exists today and that led to Medicare's Conditions of Participation (CoP) and ultimately to the very complex 21st-century system of oversight of the nation's healthcare providers.

Once Medicare was enacted in 1965, two urgent considerations presented themselves: 1) quality of care, and 2) costs. The systems designed and implemented to achieve these two purposes matched the standards and practices for care at that time, but not for long. Due to the turbulent dynamics of the healthcare industry beginning with the dramatic changes in the practice of medicine that began in the waning years of the 19th Century, to the rapid growth of the hospital industry itself, and the complications introduced by the enactment of Medicare in 1965, these two issues have been subject to constant and vigorous churning. The system evolved from the not-very-complicated procedures that focused on quality assurance and were based primarily on retrospective review in the early years of accreditation to the proactive quality-improvement approaches that are practiced today.

Avedis Donabedian, a Lebanese physician, sometimes called the father of quality assurance, conducted significant research in the relationship between quality and systems in the 1960s. He was concerned that systems management was not being taught in medical and nursing schools, and he felt that systems awareness and design were important in healthcare. However, he insisted that they be seen only as enabling tools and that the ethical dimension in the long run determined quality. He felt that the successful physician was one who understood the role of love in assuring quality of medical care—love of patient, profession, and God. Donabedian is given credit for categorizing healthcare measures by structure, process, and outcome and continued to exert influence in the quality movement until his death in 2000.

In 1971, the U.S. Congress created the Experimental Medical Care Review Organizations (EMCROs) in an attempt to reduce unnecessary utilization of physician services reimbursed through Medicare and Medicaid. By focusing on individual inpatient and ambulatory-services patients, the mission of the EMCROs was to improve not only appropriateness but also quality of care. The use of professional standards review organizations (PSROs) grew out of the EMCRO program in 1972 and was established as an amendment to Title XI of the Social Security Act. Both of these programs reviewed cases to determine whether the services being provided were necessary, whether the quality of the services met professionally recognized standards, and whether these services were provided in the most effective and economic manner possible. The general purpose of these programs was to maintain cost and medical practice control, not quality improvement. The PSROs were local in organization and the overall program was so loosely structured that there were wide variations in them that made comparison impossible. Although extensive resources were devoted to the PSRO project, it was not effective in containing increasing utilization and costs.

In the 1980s, concerns over these matters—cost containment and utilization—heated up. The continued viability of the Medicare and Medicaid programs was questioned, and action was taken to dismantle the PSRO structure and replace it with peer review organizations (PROs). The Peer Review Improvement Act of 1982 required the Secretary to contract with PROs to promote the economy, effectiveness, efficiency, and quality of services reimbursed through Medicare.

The prospective payment system (PPS) was created as the result of The Deficit Reduction Act of 1984. The purpose of this act was to contain runaway healthcare costs by reimbursing providers at a fixed rate based on diagnosis-related groups (DRGs) that would reflect resources typically used for a particular diagnosis. This payment system replaced one based on reasonable or prevailing charges. This, in turn, increased the need for oversight of quality delivery and utilization: first of all, to manage the DRG system itself—the many procedures in the many groups that make up the emerging systems; and second, to certify that the charges being made by practitioners were in line with the DRG charts. The first PROs, using randomly selected individual cases, focused on reducing admissions, were retrospective, and had punitive consequences. It became apparent to the Healthcare Financing Administration (HCFA), now known as the Centers for Medicare and Medicaid Services (CMS), and the PROs that change was necessary if the review process were to be effective in controlling costs and assuring that Medicare/Medicaid patients were receiving appropriate care. By the late 1980s, quality improvement models were being developed that addressed such things as care delivery processes and information systems.

In 1989, the PRO program shifted its focus to developing collaborative relationships with providers and creating a cooperative program to address the many complex issues that were only destined to become more complicated as time went on. In 1992, the Health Care Quality Improvement Initiative (HCQII) was created and for the first time, patterns of care and outcomes were analyzed as the means toward monitoring and improving healthcare. Under the new system, the creation of quality-improvement projects was encouraged with a focus on the analysis of patterns of excellence and error in clinical care. But evolution was relentless and HCQII became the Health Care Quality Improvement Program in 1995, which officially replaced retrospective case review with quality-improvement projects. In 2002, the PROs officially became Quality Improvement Organizations under the CMS 7th Scope of Work. The work of that scope expanded the Quality Improvement efforts and added tasks associated with Home Health and Nursing Homes.

Inevitably, the quality-review process developed electronic systems to manage and communicate procedures, processes, and results. The Hospital Quality Alliance (HQA): Improving Care Through Information was created in December 2002. Led by the AHA, the Federation of American Hospitals (FAH), and the Association of American Medical Colleges (AAMC), the HQA effort is intended to make it easier for the consumer to make informed healthcare decisions, and to support efforts to improve quality in U.S. hospitals. The major vehicle for achieving this goal is the consumer-oriented Hospital Compare website. The HQA collaborators and others support this initiative as the beginning of an ongoing effort to make hospital performance information more accessible to the public, payers, and providers of care.[3] From the health-plan side, you have CMS's Quality Assessment and Performance Improvement (QAPI) Module. In 2003, CMS published its operational guide to this web-based data collection tool to make it possible for CMS-contracted Medicare Advantage organizations to submit information on QAPI projects for evaluation and approval. This QAPI Module—designed by three quality improvement organizations—enables organizations to input their project data (via the Internet) on an online QAPI Project Completion Report. This electronic report is submitted to the Health Plan Management System database for the Medicare Advantage quality review organization to review and score and for CMS to evaluate (based on QAPI Standards) and to indicate approval of the project scores.[4]

CMS manages Medicare and Medicaid and ultimately makes decisions about which healthcare organizations may participate and receive payment for services rendered on the basis of compliance with its CoP and Conditions for Coverage (CfC). The Clinical Standards Group (CSG) in the Office of Clinical Standards and Quality in CMS is responsible for the development of quality standards for providers and suppliers in the Medicare and Medicaid programs. The activities of the CSG include:

- Directing and coordinating development of Medicare and Medicaid standards for providers, e.g., hospitals, psychiatric hospitals, skilled nursing facilities/nursing facilities (including swing beds), and intermediate care facilities for the mentally retarded and suppliers (e.g., ESRD facilities, and ambulatory surgical centers).
- Providing supportive consultation for implementation of Medicare and Medicaid standards for providers and health plans.
- Convening groups such as professional organizations, consumer advocate groups, and standards-setting organizations to discuss the content in the regulatory approach to issues.
- Coordinating Agency response to quality complaints and crises in collaboration with appropriate CMS components.
- Preparing regulation specifications, coordinating evaluation of comments, and analyzing regulation impact.
- Designing and implementing a continuous system of improvement for the CoP/CfC process.
- Developing and incorporating a strategy for using performance measures in setting standards for providers and suppliers.
- Participating in the design and development of new and innovative ways to establish performance requirements for providers and suppliers.

- Providing clinical analysis for proposed legislative changes to standards.
- Evaluating the comparability of standards of accrediting organizations to determine deemed status.[5]

Certification is supported through surveys made either by a CMS survey team or by one of the two accrediting organizations with deeming authority, HFAP or JCAHO. These surveys assess CoP compliance and evaluate whether or not an institution is providing safe and appropriate care with an emphasis on quality. They are unannounced (as of January 2006 with some exceptions), are based on random samples of actual cases, and usually last from three to five days. A regional office studies the results. If any conditions are not met, the institution may submit a plan of correction. There is no cost for a CMS survey, and the CMS regional office that has oversight of the state where the survey occurs chooses the team. The frequency is every three years for unaccredited hospitals; however, frequency depends on budget and priorities for accredited hospitals. Survey results and plans of correction are public documents.

CMS determined early on that it would provide "deeming" authority to certain accrediting bodies. That is, an organization that meets certain stipulated requirements can conduct the surveys in CMS's stead and grant accreditation, which would exempt the institutions so accredited from CMS surveys. Through 2005, CMS grants this deeming authority to two accrediting organizations: JCAHO and HFAP (an arm of the AOA).

Doubts about the effectiveness of hospital surveys in actually assuring quality of care reared its head in 1970. The question raised was how problems in the provision of care can be discovered, documented, and reported; and how well an outside team of reviewers coming to a facility over a short period of time can determine that patients are receiving the "do no harm" level of care that physicians are sworn to provide. There was also the concern of public disclosure of negative survey results by healthcare facility leadership. The Joint Commission doubted that hospitals would disclose information about problems if they felt that the information could be subpoenaed or made public. It was common knowledge that hospitals went to extraordinary means to present their institutions in the best possible, if not always the most honest, light. It was also strongly suspected that hospitals concealed embarrassing records from the surveyors.

By 1985, the focus on measuring organization and physical structure and management of administrative and clinical functions to determine performance and clinical outcomes had come under fire. There was a shift at this time that reflected Codman's original "End Result Idea" much more than the status quo of the review process in the mid-1980s. Also similar to those early days, this shift reflected what was going on in the business and industrial world at large. Two men, W. Edwards Deming and Joseph M. Juran were re-conceptualizing quality and how it could be achieved in industry. Another quality expert from industry, Philip B. Crosby, was also putting forth the idea that systems knowledge and improvements were necessary if quality were to be improved and that inspections were not necessarily useful. He also taught that statistical control was needed.

Meanwhile, public health experts were developing the ability, thanks to the advances in computer technology, to analyze large amounts of data. They were revealing discrepancies in treatment and outcomes between various geographical regions and according to factors such as income and race. This resulted in two forces: underutilization of the healthcare system by disadvantaged populations and measurement of effectiveness of healthcare spending. Out of all of this came an increasing concern about how quality in healthcare should be measured.

Deming had taught principles to improve the performance of industrial process that he called continuous quality improvement (CQI). He taught that quality was not an optimal level of performance that could be achieved by getting rid of bad operators or bad operations but that it needed to be continually made better by scrutinizing and perfecting the processes. It combined education with statistical measurement of outcomes. Future improvements were always the objective of a CQI project. Learning, cooperation, and leadership were characteristics of the environment as well as the involvement of management in the quality-focused culture.

CQI, also known as total quality management (TQM), began to invade the healthcare domains. It moved away from the inspection and punishment approach that tended to target individuals and began to focus on systems and processes. It accommodated the reality that care is provided by humans and that humans make errors, but it replaced it with a better way to go: improvement of the process rather than the punishment of error-makers. The belief was that in this way, errors would be reduced and quality of care would improve. CQI also offered the carrot of cost-control at a time when increases in the cost of healthcare were inflaming not only government and healthcare leaders but also the population in general.

A concern for quality and for the safety of patients is a given for most physicians. The opportunity to provide care for sick people is the inspiration for most of them when they choose to devote their lives to medicine. Even so, their own membership in the human race brings with it the inevitability of their sometimes erring and making bad decisions.

In 1998, at a medium-sized hospital in the Southeast in a town of about 200,000, a patient, a little boy about two years old, had ingested a household chemical and was critically ill. He happened to be the beloved nephew of one of the gastroenterologists on the medical staff, a member of an excellent and much-respected practice. This little boy received the devoted attention of some of the finest medical professionals that could be found. The members of the group joined together, determined to save the little boy's life, and he seemed to be responding to the treatment. The story of the little boy circulated all over the hospital, from the housekeeping staff all the way to the executive suites, and everyone was hoping and praying for his recovery. He began to respond to treatment and was eventually taken home with the expectation that he would continue to recover.

However, he was brought back into the hospital very soon and was clearly in crisis. Then and only then did a nurse, not a doctor, identify the problem. His heart had been severely damaged by the injury and he was critical. Attention had been so focused on the gastroenterological aspects of the case that the impact on the little boy's heart had been missed. He was evacuated to a children's hospital in a nearby city, but he did not survive. Hospital personnel grieved and sadness pervaded the hospital for weeks, but nowhere was the grief and dismay so deep as in the gastroenterology unit that had failed.

Even the most professional, dedicated, and involved medical doctors sometimes make errors and bad diagnoses and apply the wrong treatment procedures. It's important in any quality endeavor to take into account not only the devotion and dedication of the doctors but also their fallibility.

The problem is that this is not Enron. When a doctor makes a mistake, a human life is in the balance, not someone's pension plan, as significant as that is. However, measuring outcomes is not as simple as it seems. The challenge lies in creating an information capture system or database that can ensure that End Result thinking has the force and effect of assuring the best possible outcomes for most if not all patients. There's no doubt that the addition of electronic records management and the vast collection and dissemination of useful information has increased efficiency in accomplishing this objective. But it is only a tool. Making the surveys more effective must constantly be the driving force with the accrediting institutions, and this can only happen if all parties involved are willing to collaborate.

There is consensus that peer review is necessary if quality is to be assured and that review, of course, must be local. Medical staffs must discipline their own members, and they do for the most part. If a member of a medical staff is not performing in a manner that meets the standards of care that the other members expect and that accreditation requires, the physicians are the first to know. The means for dealing with such a medical staff member varies by institution; however, the likelihood that efforts to deny privileges may be the result of a personal grudge or simply territorialism complicate the disciplining of a member. Hospital administrators tend to frown on action in anything but the most serious situations for fear that the motives of the accusers are not pure and that the hospital, itself, will be litigated against. Medical staffs are not allowed to arbitrarily decide that one of their members will be denied privileges. For this reason, these cases often end up in the courts, which usually find them difficult to deal with. The very nature of the court system in America, which is to protect the rights of all, usually causes these cases to go on for years and sometimes never to be resolved.

Physicians write into their own medical staff bylaws safeguards that assure that their members have access to due process in the hope that should a case go to court nothing can be found that will overturn the decision to deny privileges. In 1971, the Joint Commission revised the standards from minimal to optimal standards and put together a committee of attorneys with expertise in hospital law to redesign fair-hearing procedures for those whose privileges have been revoked.

The problem with all of this is that it has simply increased the time and number of hearings it takes in the hospital alone to come to resolution and often very little is accomplished except bitterness between the accused and the accusers. A case is cited in *Physicians and Hospitals: The Great Partnership at the Crossroads* that at the time of the publication of the book in 1984 had run on for nine years and was still not resolved. In this case, an obstetrician/gynecologist was accused of several rules infractions for failure to use sterile surgical gloves. The very first hearing ran twelve hours over four evenings. The next one lasted for three months. And that was only the beginning. When the court ruled for the medical staff, the accused appealed, and it continued on for at least nine years. The doctor's reputation and career were ruined. Time that could have been devoted to patient care had been spent in a rancorous and very public debate. The writers of that book conclude, "The lesson for hospital medical staffs should be clear. Objective, honest peer review of the clinical performance of physicians should minimize the need for a physician whose privileges are revoked for incompetence to seek redress in the courts. If a medical staff recommends revocation to reduce competition, or because of personal dislike, due process at the hospital level won't have the magic that hospital attorneys rely upon."[6]

Managed Care

Affordable high-quality care has been an elusive dream in this country since the 1960s. The medicine of that time was pretty well captured on the Marcus Welby television show. A patient would go to the office of the primary care physician (PCP) or if necessary, the physician might even go to the patient's home. The PCP could take as much time as he felt necessary to diagnose and treat the ailment, usually sending the patient home with a prescription if the illness called for it. If the illness were severe enough, the PCP would make a referral to a specialist or suggest that the patient go to the local community hospital, a nonprofit organization. The PCP, himself, managed the case in the hospital and was in charge of any decisions that were made, using whatever resources the hospital had available—equipment, personnel, etc. Hospital management stayed out of patient care entirely.

The doctor's services and the costs related to the hospital stay were covered by some insurance plan or other, either that of the patient's employer or an indemnity plan that might have been sold by the hospital, itself.

But that was then. Today, this traditional healthcare system is gone forever and one place where it is most apparent is in the reduced level of autonomy a physician has in the matter of decision-making. Federal, state, and local healthcare rules place tight controls and constraints on how patients are followed, referred, and in some cases treated. A managed care organization may even assign and determine which PCP a patient can see, even if it is against the patient's will.

The reasons for this dramatic shift in the healthcare system are financial ones. The cost of healthcare in this country, beginning with the advent of Medicare and Medicaid, has threatened to overwhelm the economy; and finding a way to control it has necessitated change. According to David Dranove, who has been studying the economics of healthcare for many years, "in 1960, healthcare expenditures accounted for just 5.2 percent of the U.S. gross domestic product (GDP), and per capita spending on healthcare was just $149 annually (adjusted to 1997 dollars). Even so, Americans still spent 20 percent more per capita on healthcare than anyone else. Costs continued to increase through the 1960s to the point where healthcare accounted for 7.3 percent of the U.S. GDP in 1970, and per capita spending of $357 was 27 percent higher than anywhere else."[7] In 2004, healthcare expenditures in the U.S. accounted for 16% of the GDP and amounted to $6,280 per capita.

Managed care dates from the 1890s when physicians would draw up agreements to provide care for a group of patients such as unions and other organizations of workers. Eventually, very large plans emerged such as Blue Cross and the Kaiser Foundation Health Plan, established during World War II when throngs of workers were employed in Kaiser's shipyards. It became the model for creation of the health management organization (HMO) in the 1970s.

According to Dranove, managed care has, in fact, worked to hold the line on healthcare costs. He reported, "U.S. healthcare spending as a percentage of GDP peaked at 13.7 percent in 1993 and since then has stayed there or even declined slightly."[8] Though healthcare costs did spike after 2000, they then appeared to level off again as of 2004.

Is quality poorer with the departure of Marcus Welby? Patients would, for the most part, answer in the affirmative. However, the evidence doesn't seem to indicate the truth of that perception. In the first place, determining quality is difficult. In addition, patients rarely know what the outcome statistics are for a particular PCP or a Managed Care Organization (MCO), or, for that matter, a hospital. The movement toward living healthier lifestyles, making environmental awareness and improvements a priority, and enhanced preventive medical services and disease management should, theoretically, improve wellness in this country. However, it may still take some time before the causal effects of the above clearly show a direct and significant link to health improvements.

So what about certification of physicians and accreditation of hospitals? Do they assure quality? The cases that led to U.S. Senator Chuck Grassley's bill in 2004 to force changes in the way accreditation surveys are carried out would suggest that even the "gold standard" of JCAHO accreditation is not beyond scrutiny when it comes to reviewing and evaluating hospital quality-of-care provisions. The struggle to assess quality has been going on since Dr. Codman posed his End Result theory and continues until today. For example, until about 1980, quality was measured by the performance of structures and processes. Then in the 1980s, End Result theory came to the front again and measurements began to be based on outcomes; and HCFA (currently CMS) began to report mortality rates for Medicare patients. The relationship between severity of the illness and its role in measuring quality became a part of the discussions regarding measurement during that time.

Managed care has always been unpopular with patients, who complain that they do not have a PCP who takes charge of their healthcare and they don't trust the MCO to make the best decisions for them. In addition, the impersonality of the system has been a source of frequent complaint.

So is the quality poorer under the system where the PCP is no longer in the driver's seat? According to Dranove, statistics indicate that the quality is every bit as good and probably better. Spending more for healthcare did not buy better medicine. The controls that have come into the system with the introduction of managed care have, in fact, brought necessary controls, but not at the sacrifice of quality of care.

Business Steps in: NCQA and HEDIS

A coalition of large employers, foundations, and HMOs, in an effort to obtain objective information about managed care quality, created the National Committee for Quality Assurance (NCQA) in 1991. This coalition set up a system of measuring quality from a variety of angles in order to give patients information they need to shop for an MCO. The Health Plan Employer Data and Information Set (HEDIS) were created for this purpose and became the major device for reporting on HMOs. NCQA uses HEDIS to accredit health plans, and interested employers and employees may have access to a report on a particular HMO or PPO. This comprehensive, no-nonsense tool provides information that a single employer could not possibly obtain on its own. Because accreditation by NCQA is so valuable to an HMO, the effort to comply is a very strong force in the effort to assure quality. Without it, companies and individuals have little to go on when making choices as to provider. HEDIS reports include hundreds of scores and measures for each treatment area.

Unfortunately, the reports are so voluminous and data-heavy that employees tend to pass over all of this information and just focus on member satisfaction because it's the one they can easily understand. To increase their utilization, NCQA continues to improve the reports and to make them more employee-friendly.

The Premier Hospital Quality Incentive Demonstration

In July 2003, Department of Health and Human Services Secretary Tommy G. Thompson announced the Premier Hospital Quality Incentive Demonstration, a project to encourage hospitals to provide high-quality inpatient care. Thompson turned to Premier, Inc., a nationwide organization of not-for-profit hospitals because of its ability to track and report quality data for 34 measures for each of its hospitals, enabling a rapid test of incentives for high performance in several areas of quality.

Under this demonstration, hospitals were offered bonuses based on quality measures for inpatients with heart attacks, heart failure, pneumonia, coronary artery bypass graft, and hip and knee replacements. The measures included prescribing of aspirin for heart attack and bypass patients and appropriate treatment with antibiotics for pneumonia.

Hospitals would be measured on each condition, and the top 10 percent on any one of the measures would be given a 2 percent bonus on Medicare payments, with hospitals in the second 10 percent receiving a 1 percent bonus. The remainder of the top 50 percent were to be recognized for quality but would not receive a bonus.

On November 14, 2005, a press release from the CMS Office of Public Affairs announced the first results of this demonstration project. "We are seeing that pay for performance works. We are seeing increased quality of care for patients, which will mean fewer costly complications— exactly what we should be paying for in Medicare," said Mark B. McClellan, CMS Administrator.[9]

Medicare awarded $885 million during the first year of the program. Between the first and last quarters of the first year, composite scores showed the following percentages of improvement in each of the five clinical areas where quality was measured:

- From 87 percent to 91 percent for patients with acute myocardial infarction (heart attack).
- From 65 to 74 percent for patients with heart failure.
- From 69 percent to 79 percent for patients with pneumonia.
- From 85 percent to 90 percent for patients with coronary artery bypass graft.
- From 85 percent to 90 percent for patients with hip and knee replacement.[10]

The demonstration began in October, 2003, and will end in September, 2006. The press release reports that preliminary information from the second year indicates that the scores are continuing to go up with the poorest-performing hospitals improving the most.

Prescription Drugs

Before the 20th Century, the pharmaceutical industry primarily produced patent medicines. But World War II and the discovery of penicillin marked the beginning of an entirely new component in healthcare. Before that time, drugs were limited to aspirin and treatments for syphilis, diphtheria, and a few vaccines. It was only in the postwar years that the drug industry as we know it today began to emerge.

The research required to introduce a new drug has been carried on primarily at public expense with the National Institutes of Health (NIH) the granting agency. Millions of dollars are dispensed by this agency every year for the basic research that leads to new medications. Several private foundations also carry out this research through private grants. It's the application of the research that falls to the pharmaceutical companies, and the federal government even supports some of those applied research projects. The drug companies typically pay for the clinical trials of new drugs.

Until 1994, reasonable pricing clauses made it possible for the public sector to control the cost of prescription drugs; however, drug industry lobbyists were successful that year in getting the rule rescinded by preventing new drug therapies developed in the labs of the companies from getting into the hands of the government researchers. There were efforts as early as the 1960s to control drug pricing; but since that time, little has been done that was effective in impacting the rapid escalation in the costs of prescription drugs. Since the failure of the Clinton Health Care plan, annual increases have been in the double-digits.

Even so, advances in prescription medicines have transformed American lives. If only blood pressure medications and those that control cholesterol are taken into account, the extension of life as a direct result of prescription drugs is phenomenal. Any consideration of healthcare quality must take into account the role of the pharmaceutical industry and the rapid progress in the treatment of so many life-threatening diseases.

But just as senior citizens are the primary users of hospital beds, so older patients are the ones most dependent on prescription drugs; and as prices have escalated, they have moved out of the reach of many of the patients who need them most. While Medicare made hospital and physician care available to many who could not otherwise afford it, there was no such support for the life-giving, life-saving prescription drugs.

In response to this dilemma, President George W. Bush signed into law the Medicare Prescription Drug Improvement and Modernization Act of 2003 with the purpose of giving seniors and disabled persons a prescription drug benefit. Under a very complicated system, this act became a reality on

January 1, 2006, with a very chaotic introduction. It seemed that no one—not the CMS, not the insurance companies providing the plans, not the pharmacists who would be dispensing the drugs, certainly not the recipients—was prepared to implement it. Anyone on Medicare qualifies for the prescription drug benefits with the payment of a monthly premium to an insurance provider. After the payment of an annual deductible in addition to the monthly premium, a co-pay system kicks in with variations from insurer to insurer. Once an enrollee spends more than $3,600 out-of-pocket in a year for prescription medicines, Medicare and the participating drug plan will cover 95% of the costs. The plan has been criticized for working to the benefit of insurance companies and failing to improve the availability of affordable medications for many senior citizens.

The quality of the drugs being introduced into the market has often come into question, but never with more public furor than a scandal over a pain-reducing drug called Vioxx, which had been approved by the Food and Drug Administration (FDA) Office of Drug Safety. Dr. David Graham, the FDA associate director for science, reported that the FDA had ignored his studies that showed a link between the drug and heart attacks. In an interview with the American Association of Retired Persons (AARP), he reported that a clinical trial had shown that heart attack risk was four times as great in those taking Vioxx as the control group, and that an estimated 100,000 heart attacks had been due to this medication with 30,000 to 40,000 deaths. Graham put the blame on the intense advertising of the drug whereby consumers were instructed to ask their doctors for it. According to Dr. Graham, the FDA let the American people down.[11]

Dr. Graham also points out that the problem is not just a one-time situation. He says that there is an "inherent conflict of interest" because when the FDA approves a drug, they are unlikely to admit they made a mistake, and the size of study required to validate the problem costs money that the FDA does not have. He says the focus has been on getting drugs on the market as soon as possible rather than getting them out safely.

The Road Ahead

Federal agencies such as CMS coupled with private accrediting organizations like JCAHO, NCQA and HFAP; professional organizations such as the AMA, AOA, and AHA; and other responsible healthcare entities must maintain constant vigilance to make the United States healthcare system the best in the world. Sometimes, legislators must step in and provide the impetus for change such as what happened in 2004 when U.S. Senator Chuck Grassley, Chairman of the Senate Committee on Finance, introduced a bill to promote changes in the healthcare accrediting system (see chapter four for details on this bill) as the result of some very public and dramatic failures to protect patient's wellbeing and ensure the quality of healthcare. The shift from announced and planned surveys to unannounced ones is evidence that solutions can be found and that the quality revolution begun so many years ago with Dr. Codman's End Result theory will continue.

Chapter 3
The Healthcare Facilities
Accreditation Program

In the 1940s, the American Osteopathic Association (AOA) began developing an accrediting agency for institutions where their physicians were doing their rotating internships and residencies. The association wanted to be sure that these facilities were providing the level of training that met their standards for high-quality care. The work was complete in 1945, and the agency was implemented under the name Healthcare Facilities Accreditation Program (HFAP).

When Medicare was launched in 1965, only two organizations were given "deeming authority" to survey acute care hospitals on behalf of its management arm, HCFA (now CMS). Those organizations were HFAP and JCAHO. "Deeming authority," according to CMS meant that a hospital accredited by either of the associations was deemed to comply with the Medicare CoP for Hospitals as published and constantly updated by CMS. In other words, facilities accredited by either of these associations automatically qualified for reimbursement under Medicare.

Under the Clinical Laboratory Improvement Amendments of 1988 (CLIA), HFAP also received deeming authority to survey hospital laboratories as a recognized alternative to accreditation by either the College of American Pathologists (CAP) or JCAHO. The National Committee for Quality Assurance (NCQA) does not require managed care organizations (MCOs) to use a specific accrediting organization; the choice is up to the MCO. HFAP also has deeming authority for the following:

- Ambulatory Care Centers
- Ambulatory Surgery Centers
- Mental Health Centers
- Rehabilitation/Sub Acute Facilities
- Substance Abuse Centers
- Critical Access Hospitals
- Hospital Laboratories

The most recent renewal of HFAP's deeming authority came in March of 2005 and will be effective through September 25, 2009.

"The Federal government continues to recognize the HFAP as one of the premier voluntary accreditation organizations," said George A. Reuther, current HFAP director. "This renewal shows that HFAP accreditation remains a validation that a facility is meeting or exceeding the standards of quality set by CMS."[12]

While HFAP was created originally to accredit hospitals where osteopathic interns and residents worked, in recent years other healthcare institutions have increasingly used it as well. In fiscal year 2005, 23 hospitals, 2 critical access hospitals, 2 ambulatory surgical centers, and 20 ambulatory care centers applied to HFAP for accreditation. In the past four years, over 70 hospitals have employed HFAP to manage their accreditation needs for the first time. By June of 2005, 321 HFAP-accredited healthcare facilities including 137 acute care hospitals, 8 critical access hospitals, 40 behavioral health centers (mental health and substance abuse), 126 ambulatory care centers, 4 ambulatory surgery centers, and 6 rehabilitation centers were accredited by HFAP. This represents an 8.3 percentage increase in two years. In addition, accreditation approval by HFAP was in process in mid-2005 for 46 other facilities that included 18 acute care hospitals, 3 critical access hospitals, and 25 ambulatory care facilities; in addition, 7 laboratories were in the process of achieving HFAP accreditation at that time.

Hospitals are choosing this alternative to JCAHO for many reasons. In some cases, such as Russell Hospital in Alexander City, Alabama, size is a deciding factor. Russell was seeking Rural Referral Center status with JCAHO, which requires a specified level of admissions. The Russell Hospital Referral Center didn't qualify under JCAHO but it did under HFAP, so Russell made the decision to carry both accreditations. Jan Landers, Director of Quality Services and Corporate Compliance at Russell, recommends going with both accreditations if it is financially feasible.[13]

Skiff Medical Center switched to HFAP after months of nationwide research and interviews with management of HFAP accredited hospitals. Bob Campbell, Skiffs Director of Quality Management, found that "HFAP accreditation is just as credible and complete as JCAHO"; and "HFAP is more cost effective, more patient-centered and more customer-friendly." The consensus of many healthcare leaders in Iowa, Indiana and Kansas is that HFAP is extremely thorough, but fair, with clear standards that are easily understood and closely based on Medicare Conditions of Participation. Campbell shared that the hospitals Skiff surveyed were all glad they changed to HFAP.[14]

Eleven Indiana hospitals, including hospitals of the Sisters of St. Francis Health Systems, have recently switched from JCAHO to HFAP. The cost of the JCAHO survey for Reid Hospital was about $65,000 in 2002 while the cost of their HFAP survey in 2005 was $14,600.[15]

At one time, JCAHO accreditation was a given among hospital quality professionals, but that time appears to be fading. There is not a large movement away from the Joint Commission surveys, but alternatives are now being considered before decisions are made. For one thing, there are more specialized healthcare accrediting organizations available. Besides the well known alphabet soup such as JCAHO, NCQA and URAC, there are others such as the Accreditation Association for Ambulatory Health Care, the Continuing Care Accreditation Community, and COLA to name a few.

Cost also seems to be a driving factor. For a 500-bed system, for example, JCAHO's costs can run between $80,000 and $100,000.[16] This often includes hiring outside consultants as well as the loss of many staff hours at all levels to prepare for the survey. Joint Commission Resources, an affiliate of JCAHO, provides consultative and educational services to help hospitals prepare for the JCAHO survey. Consultant fees can add significantly to the overall accrediting package cost. Many hospitals are questioning whether all of this effort results in improved patient care, which is, ostensibly, the very purpose for quality reviews. Also, there is a feeling among many staff-members that this is not a user-friendly process. Ultimately, the question becomes: is accreditation worth the value received?

But some misgivings about the value of JCAHO accreditation have additional implications. A study by the General Accounting Office (GAO) from 2001 to 2004 of 500 hospitals that were accredited by JCAHO found that serious problems were often missed. The Senate Committee on Finance proposed a bill to "amend Title XVIII of the Social Security Act to revoke the unique ability of the Joint Commission for the Accreditation of Healthcare Organizations to deem hospitals to meet certain requirements under the Medicare program and to provide for greater accountability of the Joint Commission to the Secretary of Health and Human Services."[17]

In response to these complaints, JCAHO has made drastic changes in the way it conducts its surveys and how it determines whether or not an institution qualifies for accreditation. Even so, the credibility of JCAHO has been compromised and may be another reason hospitals, laboratories, et al, are considering and looking for alternatives.

Osteopathic Medicine

Doctors of Osteopathy (DOs) and Doctors of Medicine (MDs) are not very different from each other. Both must complete a four-year undergraduate degree that has a concentration in science courses, and both complete four years of basic medical education. Both may choose a specialty area following graduation from medical school such as surgery, family practice, or psychiatry and must undergo residency programs ranging from two to six years. Both must pass comparable state licensing exams and both practice in fully accredited and licensed healthcare facilities. Licensed DOs provide a full range of services from prescribing drugs to performing surgery, use current tools and technologies, and practice in both osteopathic and allopathic hospitals.

The practice of osteopathic medicine has emerged in recent years as one of the fastest growing areas in medical care. One major difference in osteopathic care is the emphasis on the inter-relationships of nerves, muscles, bones, and organs. DOs are committed to treating the whole person with a focus on primary care and prevention, diagnosis and treatment of illness, disease, and injury. More than 65% of DOs specialize in primary care, which includes family practice, internal medicine, obstetrics/gynecology, and pediatrics. However, many are also specialists in all areas such as psychiatry, cardiology, and ophthalmology.

Osteopathic medicine is people-oriented and demands dedicated and empathetic people. To be accepted for study, students must exhibit a genuine concern for others.

Osteopathic medical colleges assess this personal quality before accepting the application of a student.

The first two years in an osteopathic medical college will be devoted almost exclusively to the basic sciences. In the third and fourth years, the student will be involved in clinical work in community hospitals, major medical centers, and doctors' offices. These clinical years are spent studying general medicine; but students are also involved in research, rotating through urban, suburban, and rural settings in order to gain exposure to all areas of medicine. Relationships between body systems are emphasized in the four-year curriculum.

Following graduation, the DO will complete an approved twelve-month internship that will include rotation through hospital departments and that must include internal medicine, family practice, and surgery. Should the DO desire to specialize, he/she will spend two to six more years in additional training.

DOs are licensed to practice medicine and surgery in all fifty states with each state determining its own tests and procedures. In some states, DOs and MDs take the same licensing exams; however, in other states, the licensing exams are different.

Osteopathic physicians are committed to continuing medical education, recognizing that the study of medicine does not end with licensing. The AOA requires a specified number of continuing medical education credits every three years in order to maintain membership.

Bureau of Healthcare Facilities Accreditation

The arm of the AOA that makes decisions regarding accreditation is the Bureau of Healthcare Facilities Accreditation (BHFA), which is made up of professionals from the following healthcare fields, who are appointed by the AOA:

- Surgery
- Obstetrics
- Gynecology
- Education
- Administration
- Osteopathic manipulation
- Internal medicine
- Family Practice
- Pathology

During its meetings, usually three times a year, BHFA reviews and approves all HFAP accrediting policies, procedures, and changes in requirements. BHFA is also the final reviewer of all accrediting surveys, making certain that corrective actions are being taken by the facilities when indicated. Additionally, BHFA reviews qualifications of facilities seeking HFAP accreditation.

HFAP Surveys

Hospital Application

According to HFAP's Survey Team Handbook, a hospital applying for accreditation must meet the following basic requirements:

- Must recognize and accept specialty certification through the certifying boards of the American Board of Medical Specialties (ABMS), and the AOA on an equal basis.
- Must have been in operation for not less than three months immediately preceding the date of application for accreditation.
- Must provide professional care and hospital service on a 24-hour basis.
- Must meet all state and local licensing requirements.

The application form must be completed four months before the survey and will include scope, volume, patient population, ownership, and community clinics. It will also include information regarding location, distance from airport, a map, and a list of local hotels.

The surveys may be conducted for initial accreditation or reaccreditations, in response to complaints, in case of relocation, and in cases where there is an immediate concern about patient safety. Medicare mandated that effective January 1, 2006, surveys will be unannounced. For all HFAP accrediting surveys, the facility will have no forewarning that inspectors are coming. This new approach is intended to better determine whether or not a facility is continuously meeting Medicare's CoP and to assist hospitals to think in terms of the next patient rather than the next survey. The only facilities exempted from this are laboratories. The unannounced surveys are intended to achieve more realistic assessments of the quality of care routinely provided by institutions.

Initial HFAP applications are mailed to the qualifying facility six to eight months prior to its current accreditation (JCAHO, NCQA, CAP, etc.) expiration date. In the case of HFAP reaccreditation, the application is mailed out six to eight months prior to the three-year anniversary of its previous survey. Completed applications must be received by HFAP within 60 days after initial mailing. Once the HFAP survey application is received, acknowledged and processed, the HFAP survey team may arrive at any time before the expiration date of its current accreditation (if applicable).

The Survey Process

The HFAP survey is normally conducted during the weekdays and begins with a brief meeting with the facility administrator before the opening and introductory conference. Information such as the number of facility employees, inpatients, breakdown of medical and ancillary staff members, inpatient and outpatient census, and other health-and administrative-reporting metrics may be requested prior to the initial opening conference with the facility. Since most surveys are now unannounced, it is prudent for facilities to be able to quickly assemble such data in a relatively short period of time to provide to surveyors. Some of the areas that are surveyed include credentialing, patient safety, performance improvement initiatives, infection control, and appropriateness of patient-care priorities. It should be noted that most of the survey is spent in the patient-care areas, observing the delivery of healthcare and all support area operations.

There is always the chance that the facility's key members may not be available when the team arrives during these unannounced surveys. In such cases, the facility should have designated and knowledgeable alternates who are always ready and available as needed.

In the past, facilities have been asked to assemble documents for review prior to the arrival of the team. Now, instead, the surveyors will review pertinent facility policies while on-site.

Previously the quality improvement review session took place on the first day of the survey. Under the new regimen, this will occur on day two to allow the organization to prepare.

A list of the survey team members will be in the packet issued by the coordinator with their bio-sketches as well as an agenda and a list of documents the surveyors will need to see.

The Survey Team

A team is made up of a team captain, who is a physician; an administrator; and a registered nurse. Team captains may be osteopathic physicians or allopathic physicians. Administrator surveyors may be facility administrators or assistant administrators, and registered nurse surveyors are usually vice presidents of patient care or chief nursing officers with facility-wide background knowledge of quality assessment and performance improvement. Nurses with QAPI leadership experience are also used if their hospital background is sufficient to justify selection to the team. For larger institutions, more complex systems, or facilities that have many remote locations, additional surveyors may be used to ensure thorough coverage during the review. While performing duties, survey team members must represent the HFAP program only and cannot have any conflicts of interest such as an affiliation with the facility being surveyed. Members of the teams work part-time and on an interim basis as surveyors for HFAP. They typically hold positions in healthcare institutions commensurate with their roles on the survey team.

Optional Pre-Survey

Facilities that are requesting accreditation from HFAP for the first time may request a pre-survey consultation, which will inform the management team about requirements and identify potential accreditation problems that might need to be resolved before a full survey is undertaken. This pre-survey consultation will include a walk-through of the facility and a quick review of the facility's policy and procedure manual.

The Exit Conference

During the exit conference the team will discuss and summarize the major deficiencies, identifying any concerns involving federal, state, or local law and addressing anything that might have direct impact on the health or safety of patients or staff. This review may be followed by an open discussion; staff members may ask for guidance in responding to the deficiencies. The team will provide positive recommendations for ways to improve in the areas that show deficiencies and ways to improve performance on future surveys. The recommendations made by the survey team to the BHFA are not discussed with the facility.

The Final Report

The team captain reviews, consolidates, and submits surveyor scored worksheets to the Division of Healthcare Facilities Accreditation. All deficiencies cited in the written report must match deficiencies reported in the exit conference. The team captain will recommend approval or denial of accreditation and provide the rationale for the decision to BHFA. This report will go directly to BHFA, not to the facility being examined. The BHFA will formally notify the facility of the outcome of the survey within 60 days.

Chapter 4
The Joint Commission on the Accreditation of Healthcare Organizations

Concerns about hospital standardization first arose in the early years of the 20th Century when a major leader in the movement, Dr. Ernest Amory Codman, put forth what he called his End Result Idea, which stated that hospitals should be concerned with outcomes and their monitoring, documenting, and reporting. The ACS grew out of that movement. By the 1950s, the AMA had an accreditation program for internships and residencies and depended on the ACS to certify hospitals. Control of accreditation was hotly debated for many years, particularly between the AHA, the AMA, ACS, and the American College of Physicians (ACP). In 1950, a small negotiating team representing the four came up with a proposed agreement for a joint commission, whose board would include representatives from all of the organizations. Called at first the Joint Commission on Hospital Standardization, in the spring of 1951 it became the Joint Commission on Accreditation of Hospitals and was incorporated in Illinois in November of that year. In 1987, the name was changed to the Joint Commission on Accreditation of Healthcare Organizations (JCAHO).

A Tumultuous Start

The history of JCAHO is turbulent, and the cause for the turbulence is not difficult to discern. The four organizations along with a fifth member, the Canadian Medical Association (which later left to form its own accreditation association), were at one level or another natural enemies. Today, JCAHO is very large, bureaucratic, fragmented in some respects and nearly impossible to manage as is evidenced by the constant reinvention of itself that makes it so difficult for healthcare institutions to prepare for the surveys. Yet it is considered a premier arbiter for quality of care in the U.S. By following the history of JCAHO, we can gain some perspective about what hospitals and other healthcare organizations can do to manage this aspect of their businesses.

The standardization program instituted by the ACS in 1918 became a formalized effort of the AHA, the AMA, and the ACP in concert with the ACS to create a voluntary, private organization. When the Hospital Survey and Construction Act sponsored by Senators Lister Hill and Harold Burton (widely known as the Hill-Burton Act) was passed in 1946, the federal government relied heavily on ACS's certification.

By 1950, ACS was looking for another organization to take over the standardization program. The ACS director, Paul R. Hawley, approached the executive director of AHA, George Bugbee, who was now interested. Bugbee's members felt that the ACS did not pay enough attention to the non-medical aspects of running hospitals and had been thinking of establishing their own program. The details were worked out for the standardization program to be transferred to the AHA. However, the AMA, which had been accrediting interns and residents, feared that they might lose clinical control and sent a delegate to the AHA with an offer to either take it over or provide financial support. They felt that hospital administrators and trustees could not be trusted. Nor were they enthusiastic about a collaborative arrangement that would include the ACP.

As mounting concerns were being raised by these organizations, the ACS withdrew its offer to turn its program over to the AHA in favor of developing a collaborative arrangement that would include all four agencies. The AHA responded with a resolution to establish its own accreditation program in the hope that other professional organizations would be willing to cooperate with them. The AMA began to yield its hard-line stance, and the four groups began to meet. Those first meetings amounted to a standoff, with opposing groups arranging themselves on opposite sides of the table. The discussions, arguments, and disagreements were over who would control the new organization. The number of board seats allotted to the various member organizations was hotly debated as were other issues such as the relationship of the new organization to existing programs in the sponsoring organizations; the formulation of standards; inspections; and determination of accreditation. Ultimately, an agreement was hammered out for a Joint Commission. Even so, there was squabbling about who would have the most influence with the trustees. The AMA felt that it should, but the AHA refused to relinquish that point. The purpose of the new organization was to conduct an inspection and accreditation program, establish standards for hospital operation, and issue certificates of accreditation. The new Joint Commission on Accreditation of Hospitals was incorporated in Illinois in 1951 with equal representation from the AHA and the AMA.

Unanimity did not last long. The AMA feared that hospital administrators would be enabled to take control of clinical affairs. Some adjustments were made, such as relaxing the Joint Commission's requirements for mandatory attendance of physicians at staff meetings and the requirement that members of the medical staff be included on a hospital's board. Later, the matter of medical staff appointments became a heated issue, with the AMA resisting the requirement that professional privileges be based on certification.

An effort was made again in 1962 to eliminate the Joint Commission and make the AMA the accrediting organization. Physicians were at best lukewarm about the work of JCAHO; they were not convinced that it was improving patient care. Eventually, the AMA accepted the organization as it had originally been set up, but some adjustments were made regarding the effort to impact patient care, not just organizational structure. It was an uneasy truce as ongoing contention would demonstrate. The director of JCAHO resigned in 1964 and his parting observations suggested that JCAHO had lowered many of the standards it had established in the beginning, all having to do with the medical staff.

Under the new director, John Porterfield, the protection of interests, particularly on the part of the AMA and the AHA, were a constant in many board meetings. As other healthcare organizations began to desire accreditation, such as nursing homes, the old issues once more reared their heads. The American Nursing Home Association, for example, was uneasy about coming under the control of the hospital association and discussed the possibility of establishing its own accrediting association under the auspices of the AMA. At the same time, the AHA was working on its own program for the accreditation of extended care facilities.

Additionally, in the early 1960s, health professionals such as chiropractors and podiatrists began to lobby and litigate for hospital privileges on the basis of restraint of trade. At the same time, several malpractice cases were decided in favor of patients who had sued hospitals, rather than physicians; and in 1969, the Joint Commission was in the middle of a controversy over relationships between governing boards and medical staffs.

When Medicare gave JCAHO deeming authority following its introduction in 1965, another complicating factor was introduced—public interest. Eventually, over the objections of many in both the AHA and the AMA, public members were added to the board. Even so, the two major stakeholders fiercely held onto their majority status and no authority was relinquished. The advent of the public in the mix also meant that public awareness was beginning to be focused on the accreditation body. Public scrutiny began to heat up, and, like it or not, the AMA was sometimes forced to yield a point to protect its own image. One part of that public, the senior citizens segment, began to be vocally critical about quality of care and about the cost of care.

In the 1970s, Congress was focusing on healthcare issues and possible legislation due to exploding costs, quality concerns, and inefficiencies in every aspect of the healthcare system. The Joint Commission was called in to participate in these discussions. Some legislators wanted the federal government to take over the regulation of hospitals either directly or through a new council or commission. They were recommending the possible disbanding of the voluntary system altogether.

A compromise was worked out. Congress amended the Medicare Act in 1972 and granted to the secretary of Health Education and Welfare (HEW) the authority to carry out validation surveys of JCAH-accredited hospitals that were participating in Medicare and to conduct surveys when there were complaints that Medicare standards were not being followed.

Meanwhile, JCAH was growing. Between 1969 and 1973, total income increased by nearly 250 percent with the greatest growth in survey fees. Corporate and council members had increased their contribution by a little over 23 percent during that time, and income from this source as a percentage of total income was decreasing dramatically.

By 1975, 105 hospitals had lost their "accreditation" status because of HEW's validation surveys, mostly because of safety issues. In 1977, when the new JCAH director, John Affeldt, took over, there was discussion of abandoning the voluntary approach to accreditation of healthcare institutions and making it a function of government. The result of all of this discussion was a restructuring of the council, which included a government relations office in Washington.

In the early to mid 1980s, the question of the credentialing of medical staff was much discussed around the issues of executive committee credentialing, medical staff credentialing, or departmental credentialing. A suit was brought before the Federal Trade Commission by chiropractors and other licensed medical practitioners who were denied hospital privileges. Ultimately, non-physician practitioners won the day and were allowed to practice in hospitals and the wording "medical staff" was changed to "organized medical staff."

The number of public JCAHO board members was always carefully controlled to make certain that authority would remain in the hands of the corporate members. The public members admired the dedication and commitment of the board but were also often exasperated at the self-serving behavior of many of them.

On December 8, 1994, the credibility of JCAHO was under siege again, according to a press conference held by the AHA. The hospital association declared strong support for the Joint Commission, calling it the best means available for safeguarding the quality of the healthcare system. The AHA stated, however, that there was a crisis in confidence in the Joint Commission because of "chronic performance problems, marketing of too many add-on services and a fundamental lack of responsiveness to the needs of hospitals and their medical staffs."[18] Dick Davidson, AHA president, reported that between 15 and 20 states were looking for alternatives to JCAHO accreditation. Even though he had expressed support for the Joint Commission, he also addressed the potential withdrawal of the AMA.

The head of the AMA delegation to the Joint Commission, however, expressed confidence in JCAHO and recommended some kind of compromise instead. The AMA actually started its own physicians' accreditation program subsequent to the discussions; however, it was abandoned in early 2000. In response to all the criticism, JCAHO developed a plan (called the Action Plan) that included measurable performance objectives and timelines relating to staff responsiveness; restructuring the survey process; and surveyor credibility, monitoring, and performance. It also addressed the matter of cutting prices. In addition, it reduced the number of focused surveys and stopped charging for them while also modifying the standards manual to make it user-friendlier.

As a part of the Action Plan, an internal review of its standards as well as what is required on the part of the institutions to demonstrate compliance with the standards resulted in a reduction of the number of standards, clarification and improvement of relevance of the existing ones, and reduction of paperwork and documentation requirements on the part of the organization. Following are the revised standards-based performance areas for hospitals:

- Ethics, Rights and Responsibilities
- Leadership
- Assessment of Patients
- Management of Human Resources
- Education
- Management of Information
- Continuum of Care
- Governance
- Provision of Care, Treatment, and Services
- Management of the Environment of Care
- Medication Management
- Medical Staff
- Infection Control
- Nursing
- Improving Organization Performance[19]

The turbulent history of the JCAHO reflects the intense dedication of medical professionals to the assurance of quality of care in the country's healthcare facilities. It was an enormous undertaking at the outset and has continued to become larger and more complex as the number of people requiring care has expanded and as medical care, itself, has become more sophisticated. It's not surprising that crisis has reared its ugly head frequently during the years since Dr. Codman took the first step toward accountability in medicine. Just as JCAHO developed its aggressive Action Plan in 1994, it has constantly responded to criticisms and the many demands for improvement placed upon it by changing the way it has managed its business.

The declared mission of JCAHO is "to continuously improve the safety and quality of care provided to the public through the provision of healthcare accreditation and related services that support performance improvement in healthcare organizations."[20] Through 2005, JCAHO evaluates and accredits more than 15,000 healthcare organizations and programs in the United States. Its evaluation and accreditation services are provided for the following:

- General, psychiatric, children's, and rehabilitation hospitals
- Critical access hospitals
- Medical equipment services, hospice services, and other home-care organizations
- Nursing homes and other long-term-care facilities
- Behavioral healthcare organizations and addiction services
- Rehabilitation centers, group practices, office-based surgeries, and other ambulatory care providers
- Independent or freestanding laboratories[21]

JCAHO also provides certification status to health plans, disease-management service companies, hospitals, and other care-delivery settings that provide disease management and chronic-care services. In 2004, it added Healthcare Staffing Services (HCSS) certification for a staffing firm's ability to provide competent staffing services.[22]

As of 2005, JCAHO is overseen by a 29-member board including nurses, physicians, consumers, medical directors, administrators, providers, employers, a labor representative, health plan leaders, quality experts, ethicists, a health-insurance administrator and educators. The corporate members are the ACP, the ACS, the American Dental Association, the AHA, and the AMA. More than 1,000 people are employed in its surveyor force at its central office in Oakbrook Terrace, Illinois, and its satellite office in Washington, DC.

Areas addressed by surveyors include an organization's performance in patient rights, patient treatment, and infection control. Surveyors evaluate a facility's ability to provide safe, high quality care but also its performance on the basis of standards that measure safety and quality of patient care. Healthcare experts, providers, measurement experts, purchasers, and consumers are involved in the development of those standards.

A Concern for Oversight

In 2004, several glaring and very public instances of breakdowns in patient care in JCAHO-accredited facilities brought criticism of the organization to a fever pitch. Redding Medical Center in California had been accredited in July 2002; only a few months later, federal agents raided the hospital on the allegation that doctors had performed unnecessary heart surgeries and tests from 1999 to 2002. Some cases surfaced where healthy individuals had been subjected to open-heart surgery. Also, Maryland General Hospital in Baltimore had passed JCAHO's evaluation for accreditation twice in four years although lab-testing equipment was not functioning and hundreds of HIV tests were mishandled. In yet another case, Florida's Palm Beach Gardens Medical Center was JCAHO-accredited even though state and federal regulators were at that time investigating complaints of life-threatening infections in the heart unit.

In 2005, Dennis S. O'Leary, president of the Joint Commission, stated that being given the responsibility of deeming authority in 1965 for Medicare had come as a shock to JCAHO. "In fact, we woke up one morning and found some language in the legislation. It was a complete surprise," O'Leary told Gilbert Gaul, Washington Post Staff Writer in an interview in 2005.[23] JCAHO never lobbied for it, O'Leary insists. Government bureaucrats needed some entity to do what they had no experience doing—overseeing the quality of health care, and they were looking for an organization that could make sure that hospitals were qualified to use the millions of dollars they were getting ready to hand out.

To compound the issue, by statute Medicare officials are required to accept JCAHO's accrediting system. There is no requirement for JCAHO to re-certify its granted CMS deeming authority, meaning that CMS had no oversight of JCAHO's continued ability to perform to set standards unlike other accrediting bodies that must periodically re-certify through CMS. CMS does have the ability to indirectly check on JCAHO by performing validation surveys on facilities that are accredited by JCAHO. Validation surveys are normally performed at 5% of accredited facilities, but in recent years and due to cutbacks, validation has occurred for only one or two percent of these facilities. This percentage will increase to 5% in 2006 and beyond.

There are many arguments for and against government oversight of private programs. However, many will agree it makes sense to have regulated oversight of private entities that are charged with insuring and accrediting programs to qualify for federal healthcare reimbursements.

The U. S. Senate decided to intervene. In HR4877, Senator Chuck Grassley of Iowa, as chairman of the U.S. Senate Committee on Finance, released a report the committee had requested from the Government Accountability Office regarding the work of the JCAHO. The stated purpose: "To improve CMS's assessment of JCAHO's hospital accreditation process, we recommend that CMS modify the measure it uses to indicate how well an accreditation program detects serious deficiencies in Medicare CoPs; maximize the extent to which validation survey findings can be generalized to all JCAHO-accredited hospitals and include its survey protocol in its annual reports to Congress; and annually conduct validation surveys on a sample of JCAHO-accredited hospitals that is equal to at least five percent of all JCAHO-accredited hospitals."[24]

Shared Visions—New Pathways

In 2002, JCAHO revised its survey procedures under a program called Shared Visions—New Pathways. These new procedures had undergone extensive testing but had not yet been put into practice at the time of the Senate hearing in 2004. A test of the new approach had been conducted by then, but results were still preliminary. According to JCAHO, it wanted the process to move away from survey preparation and toward using its standards to maintain quality healthcare facilities on a continuous basis. Following are the changes:

- Reviewed and modified all standards, removing those that were redundant and making those that remained easier to understand and more relevant.
- Created a secure extranet for healthcare facilities to access for application and data transfer.
- Implemented a periodic performance review. The process requires each accredited organization to conduct a mid-cycle self-assessment against

applicable JCAHO standards; develop a plan of action to address identified areas of non-compliance; and identify measures of success for validating resolution of the identified problem areas when the organization undergoes its complete on-site survey 18 months later.

- Changed the on-site survey to be directed by the priority focus process (PFP), which aggregates organization-specific information through an automated, rules-based tool, and identifies systems and processes that are relevant to patient safety and healthcare quality.
- Implemented a tracer methodology for on-site surveys. This will permit surveyors to assess operational systems and processes in relation to the care experiences of actual patients.
- Surveyors must meet stringent new requirements including a certification exam.
- If an organization meets JCAHO's standards compliance, it will be awarded "accredited" status—there will no longer be differing levels of accreditation. No longer will facilities be given scores.
- Unannounced surveys began in January 2006.

One of the reasons for the unannounced survey is to shift the focus from preparing for a specific evaluation event to ensuring that the appropriate needs of the patients are continuously met on a daily basis. Unannounced surveys will assure that this is being maintained.

Another benefit, according to JCAHO, is the use of the accreditation process as an operational management tool and to validate the facility's continuous systems improvement efforts rather than a simple standards-compliance exercise. It will give a more accurate picture of day-to-day performance and will be more credible with outside organizations and the public; accreditation will now be a by-product of good management, according to JCAHO.

The survey can be conducted any time from January 1 to December 31 in the year it is due. In addition, random, unannounced *validation* surveys will be conducted on a five percent sample of all accredited healthcare organizations through 2008.

All reaccrediting surveys will occur between 18 and 39 months from the previous full survey. For example, Laboratory Service reaccreditation surveys must be conducted every 24 months, and the survey must be conducted within 6 months of expiration of the last full survey.

The following surveys will not be conducted unannounced:

- Initial surveys including those conducted under the early survey policy
- Disease-specific care reviews (unannounced within 45 days either before or after the organization's anniversary date)
- Where not feasible – certain agencies are given a five-day notice (e.g., Bureau of Prisons, Department of Defense)
- Foster care programs
- Immigration facilities
- Office-based surgery practices with less than 1,500 annual visits
- Very small programs
- Option 2 and Option 3 Periodic Performance Review surveys
- Organizations have ten "blackout dates" per year.

The Survey

What to expect: On the morning of the survey, the healthcare organization's PFP summary report, the survey agenda, and the biographies of surveyors will be posted to JCAHO's secure extranet site. When surveyors arrive, there will be a one-hour Surveyor Arrival and Preliminary Planning Session. The organization will have time to review the PFP at this time. The organization should be prepared to demonstrate to the surveyors the means it uses to help people contact JCAHO to resolve quality or safety concerns.

The Survey Team

The teams typically are made up of a physician, a nurse, and a hospital administrator, all who have management-level experience in health-care organizations. If the volume or range of services of a hospital calls for it, additional surveyors with expertise in particular areas may be added. The Joint Commission has 500 surveyors who work full-time for JCAHO. These surveyors have extensive training for their roles before they ever go into the field. Continuing education is also required in order to assure that the surveyors are up to date on quality-related evaluations.

The team will be in the facility for several days observing, interviewing patients and staff, and looking at documents. Much of their time on location will be spent in patient units, observing care as it is being administered. They may also track a specific patient in-person and through medical records to measure the effectiveness of the systems and processes as they pertain to patient care. They don't make instant judgments but rather pay attention to what is going on, how well the tasks are being performed, and if possible, recording outcomes for a variety of patients and illnesses. The surveyors will have a set of guidelines and will be scoring them in order to ultimately make judgments about standards compliance.

The Evaluation

Team members bring their own background and expertise to the project, so evaluation tasks are divided up along those lines to the extent possible. Even so, team members work together in compiling their findings when they are ready to draw conclusions about the overall performance of the facility.

After the survey is completed, JCAHO will assess how well the hospital meets the standards in the accreditation manual. This assessment, along with related performance considerations, normally determines the category of accreditation. Once accredited, the facility must maintain compliance with all standards for the three-year cycle until reaccreditation.

Fees

In 2006, the fee for the Joint Commission's on-site full survey will increase by 5 percent. This will amount to an overall increase of less than 1 percent in fees paid by accredited organizations, thanks to a new billing approach that will also be introduced in 2006, called subscription billing. What was previously called the "survey fee" will be split into four separate payments—three accreditation fees of approximately 20 percent of the previous three-year fee plus an on-site fee amounting to approximately 40% that will not be billed until the time of the survey. The on-site fee is the portion that will increase by 5% in 2006 with no increase in the annual billing amount. Annual base rate fees for any other on-site surveys will see no increase. In case of a review hearing panel, that fee will increase from $1,500 to $2,500.

Chapter 5
TÜV America, Inc.

On December 12, 2005, TÜV America issued a press release announcing that CMS had begun formal evaluation of an application by TÜV Healthcare Specialists (TÜVHS) for full deeming authority. If approved, this would be the first new accreditation service for U.S. hospitals since the establishment of Medicare and the granting of deeming authority to JCAHO and HFAP in 1965. According to Rebecca Wise, CEO of TÜVHS,

> Choice and competition are the hallmarks of a free market, can you think of a more profound impact on our lives than healthcare? Yet there is a much higher chance of you getting the wrong dosage of medicine in a hospital than there is of a manufacturer putting the wrong chip on a circuit board. It's a failure of the system, not the people....Healthcare providers are so inundated with compliance and regulatory obligations that they can't spare the resources to pursue quality as a separate "project." Quality management needs to be

> seamless and self-regulating. That is the advantage of
> ISO 9001 versus all other quality initiatives. [25]

Some hospitals and medical practices currently use ISO 9001. However, at this time, TÜV does not have deeming authority, so hospitals still must qualify for Medicare and Medicaid reimbursement through the usual channels. Those hospitals may choose to take advantage of the state audit coordinated by CMS rather than undergoing an accreditation review by JCAHO or HFAP. ISO certification will be a precondition of TÜVHS's accreditation program for hospitals and healthcare organizations, provided deeming authority is granted.

TÜV Healthcare Specialists (THS), headquartered in Cincinnati, OH, is a healthcare management systems evaluation, accreditation, and training company. THS has developed an integrated accreditation program based on ISO 9001 for hospitals in the United States called National Integrated Accreditation for Healthcare Organizations (NIAHO). The International Organization for Standardization (ISO) is based in Geneva, Switzerland. Founded in 1946, this international organization was responsible for developing the first international standards for manufacturing, trade, and communications. Initially published in 1987, ISO 9001 defined the components that are required for a quality management system and detailed the necessary requirements for the quality function of industries. The body that represents the United States is the American National Standards Institute (ANSI) in the ninety-country organization. Over half a million companies worldwide claim ISO 9001 certification, 50,000 in North America. ISO 9001 certification signifies a commitment to continual improvement in quality.

ISO 9001:2000 is a revision that incorporates improvements in three areas:

- Creating a common structure based upon a process model.
- Creating a method to demonstrate continual improvement and customer satisfaction.
- Developing metrics to determine how effectively internal processes are working with a focus on improving results.

Reflecting TÜV's management philosophy of continual quality improvement, the ISO Technical Subcommittee is at work developing the next ISO standard.

The Audit

When a hospital applies to TÜV for an audit, the healthcare consultants will meet with the hospital's representatives and determine what needs to be done to prepare for it. An audit plan will be drawn up that will include a description of the work to be performed and what staff will be required to conduct the audit.

The length of the audit will be determined by the size of the hospital. If several areas are performing identical tasks, sampling techniques will be used. The auditors will first tour the facility and observe. The second phase will be interviews of employees working at various levels. The third will be a review of documentation and evaluation of quality records.

HIPAA Audit

- Review of Privacy Practices
- Assessment of Administrative, Physical and Technical Safeguards
- Review of HIPAA Forms and Documentation
- Review of Complaint Process

Corporate Compliance Plan

- Review of Compliance Plan
- Review of Written Policies & Procedures
- Review of Risk Areas
- Review of Training and Education Documentation
- Review of Auditing and Monitoring Procedures

The auditors will evaluate the institution's quality management system and compare it to the ISO 9001 standard; they will also compare practices and determine whether or not they reflect the quality documentation. In addition, the quality management system will be compared to the institution's business objectives, strategies, and vision statement. Auditors will look beyond the numbers and search for ways to increase efficiency, process effectiveness, and quality. TÜV calls its auditing approach "Insight Auditing."

In the closing meeting, problems that have been discovered will be reviewed and recommendations regarding accreditation shared. If accreditation is not recommended, the audit team will confer with the organization's leadership and work with them on follow-up actions. The only way an institution can fail is if it decides not to proceed or cannot correct areas of nonconformance.

History of TÜV

Independent TÜVs (Technischer Überwachungsverein, English translation: Technical Inspection Association) were founded in the 1870s by the German steam boiler industry in the interest of public safety. Beginning with only 43 members, it expanded quickly, reflecting the rapid advancement of technology during that time. As industries proliferated and expanded, the regulating organization also grew and included many electrically powered devices as well as diesel engines, etc. Into the latter decades of the 20th Century, the

TÜV name meant public safety, quality, and environmental protection in Bavaria. Changes in trade practices in Europe in the 1990s made it possible for TÜV to begin to compete nationally and internationally and led to the organizing of TÜVs in Europe; and in 2004, TÜV Süddeutschland became the TÜV SÜD Group. There are many TÜV organizations in the world, but the largest one is TÜV SÜD.

TÜV America Inc. was founded in 1987 as a subsidiary of the TÜV SÜD Group. TÜV America's business is international safety testing and certification services, and it now employs more than 200 experts. Many hospitals in the United States are already employing TÜV Healthcare Specialists to obtain ISO certification in addition to maintaining the CMS approvals necessary to receive Medicare reimbursement.

According to TÜV Healthcare Specialists, hospitals need to adhere to the ISO 9001 Management System standard if they are to truly improve health care. They suggest that management systems can be dramatically improved, which will lead to improved patient safety and operational performance, according to them. The NIAHO program is the first one to provide hospital accreditation based on ISO 9001 certification.

Chapter 6
Making Accreditation Choices

Without reimbursement from Medicare, most hospitals cannot survive. So the very first consideration when it comes to accreditation and certification is the reimbursement issue. However, if that were the only consideration, all hospitals would turn to CMS, since it provides surveys and certification without fees.

However, there are many other matters to be considered. An important one is community confidence. Hospitals make certain the news media in their community get the press release when accreditation is awarded. JCAHO even sells a "We are accredited" banner for hospitals to display. While community leaders and even private citizens may not understand exactly what the issues are in accreditation, they do respond to the publicity. If there's anything they want in the hospital that is responsible for their welfare when they are ill, when they are most vulnerable, it is the security of knowing they are getting the best possible care; and that magical word, "accreditation," communicates that. The more competitive the environment, the more important this facet of accreditation becomes. If the hospital across town is accredited, then this hospital must also be accredited in order to hold onto market share.

In some cases, liability insurance premiums are reduced if a hospital is accredited. Balancing the high cost of liability insurance against the cost of accreditation figures into the decision to accredit/not accredit. In addition, the ability to attract medical staff is strengthened by accreditation. When a physician is making a choice about affiliation with a hospital, he/she will take accreditation into account. Administrators are mindful when making budgetary choices that while reimbursement follows the patient, the patient follows the physician. To hold onto market share, the hospital must attract the best physicians possible and maintain good working relationships with them. If accreditation is important to the medical staff, then administration will strive to accommodate that preference.

In the past, accreditation meant being evaluated on the basis of outcomes, organizational structure, and equipment and processes, and having the grade report made public, which has led in many cases to elaborate and costly preparations for an upcoming survey. There has been a strong feeling, especially among medical staff members and hospital administrators that this dance between the facility and the accrediting organization has not led to an improvement in quality of care. However, the accreditation process itself has evolved rapidly in the past few years and has become a significant provider of instruction and consultation on the improvement of quality. This change has come about as a result of the interaction between hospital administrators, medical staffs, hospital employees, and surveyors. Today, the relationship between the accrediting entity and the facility being surveyed is a collaborative one. The objective of a survey is no longer just to determine whether a facility is performing according to a set of standards but to advance the institution's own effort to practice and improve the quality of care. When choosing an accreditation agency, the hospital will be sensitive to the quality of the education and consulting provided by that agency. If a facility decides to forgo the surveys by an accrediting body, which often provides the impetus to improve quality and increase training and education, it should put an effective substitute in its place.

Hospitals deal in life and death. Dread of a disaster with a patient and the publicity, anguish, and liability that come with it are never far from the minds of the patient-care staff in a hospital. No matter how dedicated, qualified, and professional the doctors, nurses, technicians, etc., most hospitals have in their histories at least one such incident and usually more where care was either compromised or was perceived to be compromised and where the consequences were painful. For example, in a medium-sized hospital on the west coast a few years ago, a lung-cancer patient died during surgery. The surgeon was one of the most respected physicians in the area—known not only for his skill as a surgeon but also for his commitment to his patients. In the course of the surgery, an artery was nicked. It was a minor injury and was quickly contained. However, the cancer was more extensive than the team had anticipated, so as lead surgeon, he called for a consultation by the team once the minor wound had been stabilized. The team discussed two options: 1) just close the chest since the lung could not be saved, or 2) remove the lung. The lead surgeon wanted to remove the lung because he felt that it would give the patient a few more years, and he felt that it could be taken out successfully. Some of the other team members disagreed, but they accepted his decision. As it turned out, the malignancy had invaded the heart wall, and the attempt to remove the growth opened a hole; it could not be repaired, and the patient died. Because of the extent of the unforeseen invasion of the malignant tissue into the heart, he would not have lived long even if the chest hadn't been opened up.

CMS as well as local authorities in this town required that an "unexpected occurrence" in the course of a surgery be reported; so the surgeon, through the hospital, reported to the local coroner that the artery had been nicked. Although that event was not reported as causative, the death of the patient was also reported. The local newspaper regularly monitored these reports to the coroner, looking for an exciting news story about the hospitals and in a headline the next day announced that a surgeon had killed a patient in the operating room of the hospital by nicking an artery. Efforts to set the record straight were futile. Many of the patients who were scheduled for surgery at the hospital called and canceled. The public relations office was inundated with callers. Even though the medical community understood what had happened and that the newspaper did not report the whole or even the true picture, the image of the hospital was tarnished; the quality of the care it provided was now suspect; many of the doctors who had been bringing their patients there were encountering resistance; and referrals to physicians on staff fell off. Hospital administrators must do whatever is in their power to protect the image of the hospital, and that factor figures in the accreditation choice.

Risk management and risk reduction should also be taken into consideration when making these decisions. Perhaps the most important position in a hospital is risk manager. He or she is the one who feels most heavily the burden of the potential for disaster. Most accreditation organizations actively participate in training and education to continually improve quality, which is the most important factor in preventing such things as an accident in surgery that *does* have fatal consequences, or the removal of the wrong limb as happened in a Florida hospital a few years ago, or open-heart surgery on healthy patients as happened in a California hospital. Sometimes, a visiting team of surveyors looking at the same thing can see weaknesses that even a vigilant risk manager might miss.

Last but not least in deliberations regarding accreditation/no accreditation or choosing between one accrediting organization and another is attracting payer contracts. It's the hospital administrator who is usually responsible for persuading corporations and organizations to contract with the hospital for delivery of services to employees. Hospital X, located in Ohio, was responding to the pressures that managed care was putting on it in the mid-1990s by developing contractual arrangements with local businesses (primarily PPOs) to provide comprehensive healthcare services. The hospital had, unfortunately, lost its edge in labor/delivery. In negotiations with a major corporation in the region that had a very large staff, employees were called together to discuss the contract their management team was arranging. When employees learned that the contract was with hospital X, there was an outcry because of the poor reputation of the labor/delivery unit. Employees in most companies are of childbearing age, as was the case with this company's task force. The employees refused to go to this hospital for the delivery of their babies and protested so loudly that their managers had no alternative but to back out of negotiations and contract with another hospital. While accreditation wasn't the issue in this case, it does play a part in negotiations for payer contracts. CEOs are very mindful that these decisions will be scrutinized carefully by their employees and will do everything in their power to work out contracts with healthcare institutions that pass muster.

For some institutions, especially smaller ones, cost plays an important role in their decisions regarding accreditation. Ed Lovern reported in his article "Opting out: For some systems, JCAHO's accreditation cost is more than its benefit,"[26] that the John C. Lincoln Health System in Phoenix had chosen to be surveyed by the Arizona Department of Health Services on behalf of CMS. As reported by Lovern, Dan Coleman had written a letter to the president of JCAHO telling him, "We have concluded that the cost of participating in the JCAHO process is out of proportion to the value received." Lovern also reported that a system in Missouri had made the decision to quit using JCAHO accreditation about a year earlier.

Lovern reported that Russell Massaro, JCAHO's executive vice president in charge of accreditation operations, had told him that the reason some hospitals were choosing not to accredit was the cutbacks they were experiencing and the increasing trend to scrutinize all expenditures more carefully. Coleman estimated that the 2001 survey of Lincoln would come to $86,000. Oryx, JCAHO's outcomes reporting tool, would cost another $24,000, according to Lovern. Coleman told him that there would be other costs such as conferences to stay current with JCAHO's constantly changing standards.

At an education program sponsored by Pacific Health Services Group and reported in a special supplement to its newsletter, *Briefs Focus*, November 30, 2001,[26] representatives of each of those organizations presented the three alternatives for certification/accreditation. Mark Crafton, Director of State Relations for JCAHO was its presenter. He told the participants that the average cost for a survey across the country at the time was $23,000 exclusive of indirect costs. George Reuther, Director of HFAP, reported that the average cost for the HFAP survey was $20,000 to $25,000. While the cost of a survey may seem the same, HFAP had and continues to have little to no add-on fees while JCAHO had and continues to have many. These add-on fees must be taken into account when calculating total costs.

State Surveys (CMS)

The State Surveys offered by CMS will meet the first requirement—reimbursement. However, in competition with other hospitals that are accredited, being certified by CMS does not bring with it the marketing power of the "We are accredited" slogan. The confidence of the community is vulnerable especially if a competing hospital is accredited. The reduction in liability premiums is lost and must be balanced against the cost of accreditation. In order to achieve continuous quality improvement, the hospital, itself, will need to invest in educational programs and the cost of consultants may need to be added to the operational costs. These costs must be calculated in the decision to walk away from accreditation. More importantly, some payer contracts will probably be lost.

Even so, some hospitals are opting for certification with CMS. For example, one of the John C. Lincoln Health System hospitals, 239-bed John C. Lincoln Hospital–North Mountain, Arizona, will be inspected by the Arizona Department of Health Services to qualify for Medicare reimbursement. Both John C. Lincoln hospitals had previously been accredited by JCAHO.

Joint Commission on Accreditation of Healthcare Organizations

Joint Commission accreditation certainly brings with it the assurance of Medicare reimbursement. Long considered the "gold standard" for accreditation in healthcare, it engenders community confidence. While patients and potential patients may not understand what it means, they do respond to the publicity that goes along with a passing grade from JCAHO. Doctors have a somewhat better understanding of accreditation by JCAHO than do patients and many will choose to practice in a hospital that has this hallmark rather than one that does not. Some sought-after specialists may migrate to JCAHO-accredited hospitals due to brand name alone, even if they are not necessarily convinced that the survey process improves patient care. In addition, their own credibility may suffer if they choose to practice in a non-accredited facility, and that may affect their long-term careers.

For insurance rating, hospital accreditation by JCAHO is good. There are varying forms of hospital certification and accreditation; hospital's that receive reviews from outside agencies of their quality processes will generally receive good malpractice insurance premiums.

JCAHO has a very large and impressive education and consultation program. Especially with the shift to unannounced surveys, the work of JCAHO in continuous quality improvement is important to a hospital. Now, preparation for a survey must be ongoing since the institution does not know when it will occur. Putting on a best face means to be continually prepared to be surveyed, and JCAHO offers superior education and consulting services.

Cost is the most-often-given reason for not choosing JCAHO for accreditation. Some hospitals, such as two rural hospitals in Carraway Methodist Health System in Birmingham, Alabama, may be forced to forgo JCAHO accreditation because the cost has become prohibitive, says Assistant Administrator Michael Sheffield. Another objection is what JCAHO calls its "tailored survey policy," which requires all services a hospital provides to be surveyed by them if the hospital is to be accredited, even assisted-living facilities and school-based health centers. Gary Duncan, president and chief executive officer of the 269-bed Freeman Health Center in Joplin, Missouri, says that this is the reason his hospital dropped JCAHO accreditation.[27]

As mentioned previously, the fee for the Joint Commission's full on-site survey has increased by five percent in 2006. This will amount to an overall increase of less than one percent in fees paid by accredited organizations, thanks to a new billing approach called subscription billing. What was previously called the "survey fee" will be split into four separate payments—three accreditation fees of approximately twenty percent of the previous three-year fee plus an on-site fee amounting to approximately forty percent of the previous fee that will not be billed until the time of the survey. It is only the on-site fee that will increase by five percent with no increase in the annual billing amount. Annual base rate fees for any other on-site surveys will see no increase. In case of a Review Hearing Panel, that fee will increase from $1,500 to $2,500.

While JCAHO remains the biggest and best known of the accreditation organizations, its attraction for purposes of image and prestige has been somewhat damaged recently by several instances where hospitals with egregiously dangerous practices had recently been surveyed and accredited. These situations became very public when the FBI intervened and closed one of the hospitals in California. The publicity surrounding the failures of JCAHO was intensified when Senator Chuck Grassley, chairman of the U.S. Senate Committee on Finance, sponsored a bill to authorize CMS to remove JCAHO's deeming authority. In response, JCAHO underwent a major revision called Shared Visions–New Pathways that included unannounced surveys that began in January 2006.

Whether the revamping of JCAHO will assure that it remains the premier healthcare accrediting body remains to be seen. The application of TÜV America in December of 2005 for deeming authority has the potential for changing the situation. If TÜV is approved, there may be others lined up to challenge JCAHO's ownership of the market.

Healthcare Facilities Accreditation Program

The accrediting program of HFAP has been the only alternative to JCAHO as an independent and CMS-approved hospital accrediting body since the enactment of Medicare and Medicaid in 1965. Designed originally to accredit hospitals where its DO physicians were interns and residents, in recent years it has been chosen by some allopathic hospitals as an alternative to JCAHO. Some reasons given include the user-friendly nature of the surveys; the straightforward fees that do not require costly add-ons; and its unblemished history as compared to JCAHO.

As an accrediting body that assists healthcare facilities to qualify for federal health program reimbursements, HFAP and JCAHO are mutually capable. In some communities, the term JCAHO has no particular significance. It may have relevance and significance in a competitive market, where the JCAHO-accredited institution may make the community aware that its JCAHO accreditation is considered the "gold" standard. But in reality, and for purposes of liability insurance, the insurers typically are only concerned that the institution is accredited.

The lack of HFAP brand recognition compared to JCAHO may have an effect on recruiting some specialists. While accreditation is certainly an important factor, it is not the only one. Hospitals must look at all the factors that affect the decision of a physician to apply for membership on the medical staff.

How much does it cost to maintain quality in a rapidly changing field like medicine? This factor must be considered when making these choices. The training and consulting of JCAHO, although costly, may be considered high quality. However, JCAHO is not the only source for state-of-the-art training. There are many other organizations that specialize in training for the maintenance of quality in medicine. The institution, itself, may be able to hire and train personnel who will review, monitor, and ensure compliance with quality care standards for patients. When choosing an accreditation option, these matters must be factored in. Risk management and risk reduction are directly tied to the continuous quality improvement program of a hospital, as are the skills of the persons responsible for these two functions.

In some markets, what applies to community perception may also apply to payer contracts. If community perception is impacted by the marketing efforts of a competitor that is accredited by JCAHO, community contracts may also be affected.

The following table provides a comparison of how the major hospital accrediting options stack up against important factors that should be considered. The weighing and scoring of these factors were not scientifically measured; they were qualitatively scored based on reviewed literature.

Comparison Table			
Factors	**CMS**	**JCAHO**	**HFAP**
Medicare Reimbursement	*Excellent*	*Excellent*	*Excellent*
Community Confidence	*Good*	*Good*	*Good*
Liability Insurance Reductions	*Good*	*Good*	*Good*
Attracting Medical Staff	*Good*	*Very Good*	*Good*
Survey Training/ Assistance	*Not Good*	*Very Good*	*Very Good*
Survey Process	*Good*	*Good*	*Excellent*
Accreditation Image	*Good*	*Very Good*	*Good*
Risk Management/ Reduction	*Neutral*	*Neutral*	*Neutral*
Private Payer Contracts	*Good*	*Excellent*	*Very Good*
Cost	*Excellent*	*Not Good*	*Very Good*

Table Analysis

As for **Medicare reimbursement**, there is no difference in the three. The state provided CMS certification survey provides the same level of healthcare reimbursement that accreditation does. However, **community confidence** may be compromised with only CMS certification, particularly if there is a competing institution that is accredited. Because JCAHO has long been the "gold standard," it will have an edge over other types of certification/accreditation only if competing institutions raise the issue. But in the minds of most laypersons, sanctioned and approved accreditation by a reputable organization is good enough, with little concern over whether it's JCAHO or HFAP awarding the designation.

A non-accredited facility may be penalized with high **liability insurance premiums**. In fact, the hospital's legal representation may require that it be accredited. Whether a distinction will be made on the basis of whether JCAHO or HFAP accredits will vary from institution to institution, but it is a consideration that needs to be investigated before a decision is made about accreditation.

Medical Specialists who are concerned about advancing their status and career path will probably choose to affiliate with highly reputable and accredited institutions. It just happens that most large, non-rural U.S. based hospitals are accredited through JCAHO.

Of the three organizations listed, JCAHO offers extensive accreditation **training and consultation**. However, it is costly, and it is arguable whether all the training material offered is actually needed and beneficial. It's also possible that the accrediting preparation and training materials can be obtained in ways other than JCAHO affiliates. There are many well-respected organizations that offer the courses and consultation that will enable an institution to protect itself against risks and to continually improve its quality of care.

Some institutions hire or contract with accrediting experts to support their facilities, while others send staff members to extended courses who in-turn provide in-house training to facility staff.

HFAP boasts a "customer-focused" **survey process** that is not disruptive to normal operations. HFAP strives to accomplish the accrediting process in the most personable, flexible, and accessible manner possible.

Beginning with the application process and continuing on through the on-site survey, HFAP has been described by hospital officials as flexible and educational, with a responsive and helpful staff.

On one occasion, BHFA, the accrediting decision body for HFAP, scheduled and called to order a special session to expedite Hillsdale Community Health Center's accreditation status in time so that they could complete their CMS Rural Referral Center application before the deadline. The Hillsdale President and CEO felt that JCAHO would never have scheduled a special meeting for this purpose. Hillsdale management personnel also expressed their appreciation for the cooperative and supportive approach of the HFAP surveyors as opposed to being purely judgmental.

The management of one Belleville, Illinois, hospital reported that while the HFAP survey was thorough and probing, the surveyors conducted the survey in a professional, friendly, and non-confrontational manner that was not typical of their prior JCAHO survey experience.

At a medical center in Philadelphia, Pennsylvania, managers reported how much they learned from the HFAP survey team. AOA and HFAP represented themselves as a very knowledgeable and customer-friendly accrediting body.

The **image** of the healthcare facility depends on many things. JCAHO has been used often to polish an institution's image. However, it takes only one disaster where media reports that a patient's life or well-being has been endangered, and the prestigious appellation is not of much use. From a brand perspective, JCAHO is well known and widely dispersed. But there doesn't appear to be any supporting evidence that the image of facilities accredited through HFAP have been tarnished. **Risk management** and a focus on continuous quality improvement are the best ways to avoid these occurrences, not only for purpose of preserving the mission of the facility but also to hold onto market share. On the surface, JCAHO seems to provide the best means to do that. However, it has been proven several times recently that the facts don't necessarily match the perception. Several hospitals and laboratories that were accredited by JCAHO, many of them recently, were found to be woefully lacking. In all of those cases, the welfare and in some cases, the lives of patients were put in jeopardy. HFAP does not have this history. Though it is not as well known, being accredited by HFAP may, in the long run, be the safest way to protect the hospital's image. Risk management could perhaps be better served by education/consulting on continuous improvement directed by the healthcare facility rather than an outside accrediting body.

It will be difficult for a healthcare facility to attract **payer contracts** if it is not accredited. Company CEOs and staff want assurances that the care they receive from a chosen hospital is the best available, and that's what accreditation says to them. Because HFAP is not as well known as JCAHO, there might be some concerns about its reputation in some markets, but in others, management and employees just want to know that the institution is monitored and accredited to ensure it provides superb care.

From a **cost** perspective, accreditation from CMS through the state has no associated fees. However, facility preparation may have some direct and indirect costs associated with it. There are direct fees associated with accreditation through either JCAHO or HFAP; however there still appears to be a larger total cost associated with the JCAHO process than with HFAP.

Chapter 7
Conclusion

Fluidity in the accrediting of healthcare institutions is likely to increase rather than decline in the immediate future, especially if CMS grants TÜV deeming authority, which may open the floodgates for other quality initiatives to apply. Even if CMS denies TÜV's application, the pressures put on JCAHO by the Senate and by the very public disclosure of its failures will continue to create management challenges for administrators, medical staffs, and governing boards. With more accrediting choices, careful scrutiny of internal operations will be necessary to make the best decisions for your facility. It's certainly true that understanding every aspect and having at hand in-depth knowledge about how each part of the business operates will be even more crucial than ever in managing this part of the business. The people who answer to the CEO and who are in charge of the various departments such as nursing and facility-management will need to be reliable and dedicated. The CEO will need to trust their knowledge, commitment, and evaluations more than ever.

The advent of unannounced surveys changes everything. No longer can a hospital rely on last-minute preparations to pass muster with the surveyors. Adjusting to the new reality of every-day readiness will call for changes in procedures and processes. More frequent reports will be necessary. Employees may need to be added to be sure there will be knowledgeable, prepared people available when the knock comes on the door. Constant and continuous preparation for surveys has the potential for improving quality of care in all institutions if it's taken seriously. It is designed to avoid some of the disasters of recent years such as the open-heart surgery on healthy patients that was occurring in a hospital in California or the bungled HIV analyses that occurred in a Maryland hospital. While the new surveys may cause consternation in some areas of the hospitals, the risk managers will probably welcome the help in keeping the departments vigilant.

The best accrediting approach will depend on your institution's needs. How important is accreditation to community perception of your hospital? How much competition do you have for market share? Will your competitor(s) compare your accreditation status to theirs to influence doctors and patients? How important is cost? Do JCAHO's fees and add-ons put an undue burden on your equipment and personnel resource allocation budget? What will be the impact on payer contracts and on liability insurance if you forgo accreditation by HFAP or JCAHO? How does your medical staff feel about change? What will it cost to obtain the training and consultation necessary to achieve continuous preparedness? Will you outsource or use internal resources to provide the accrediting training and education needs for your facility? These and other factors must be considered when making your accrediting choices. Once you've answered these questions, you should then look at what each of the accrediting institutions has to offer in the way of acceptable benefits for your facility.

The bottom line is there are alternatives to JCAHO that should be considered. HFAP is one such choice; facilities that have switched from JCAHO to HFAP rave about its uncomplicated survey process and assistance approach, its compliance with the CMS rules, and its lower survey costs as compared to those of JCAHO.

Bibliography

Agency for Healthcare Research and Quality. "Medicare's Hospital Bill." *AHRQ News and Numbers*, November 16, 2005.

Brauer, Carl M. *A History of the Joint Commission on Accreditation of Healthcare Organizations*. Lyme, Connecticut: Greenwich Publishing Group, Inc., 2001.

CMS. "Conditions for Coverage (CfCs) & Conditions of Participations (CoPs)" http://www.cms.hhs.gov/CFCsAndCoPs/ (Downloaded September 18, 2006.)

CMS Office of Public Affairs, "Medicare Demonstration Shows Hospital Quality of Care Improves with Payments Tied to Quality." Press Release, November 14, 2005.

Dranove, David. *The Economic Evolution of Healthcare: From Marcus Welby to Managed Care*. Princeton, NJ: Princeton University Press, 2000.

Gaul, Gilbert M. "Accreditors Blamed for Overlooking Problems," washingtonpost.com, July 25, 2005.

Goozner, Merrill. "What Went Wrong?" *AARP Bulletin*, January 2006.

Government Accounting Office. *Medicare: CMS Needs Additional Authority to Adequately Oversee Patient Safety in Hospitals,* July, 2004.

"HFAP Survey Earns Facility Referral Status: Stays with JCAHO, Now Has Two Certifications." *HealthCare Benchmarks and Quality Improvement:LookSmart,* Oct, 2003.

Hodgson, Patricia, and Duncan Yagge, Eds., *Physicians and Hospitals: The Great Partnership at the Crossroads.* (Based on the Ninth Private Sector Conference, 1985.) Durham, NC: Duke University Press, 1985.

House Bill #HR4877.

Joint Commission on Accreditation of Healthcare Organizations. "What is the Joint Commission on Healthcare Organizations?" (Downloaded September 18, 2006.) http://www.jointcommission.org/AboutUs/joint_commission_facts.htm

Lovern, Ed. "Opting out: For some systems, JCAHO's accreditation cost is more than its benefit." *Modern Healthcare,* June 18, 2001.

Medicare+Choice Quality Review Organizations for the Centers for Medicare & Medicaid Services (CMS), *QAPI Module Operational Guide, Version 1.0.* April 2003.

"QI Professionals Take Harder Look at Alternatives to JCAHO Accreditation." *Healthcare,* September, 2003.

Endnotes

[1] Agency for Healthcare Research and Quality, "Medicare's Hospital Bill."

[2] Carl M. Brauer, *A History of the Joint Commission on Accreditation of Healthcare Organizations*, p. 21.

[3] http://www.hospitalcompare.hhs.gov

[4] QAPI Module Operational Guide, Version 1.0. Prepared by the Medicare Choice Quality Review Organizations for the Centers for Medicare & Medicaid Services (CMS).

[5] http://www.cms.hhs.gov/CFCsAndCoPs/

[6] Patricia Hodgson and Duncan Yagge, Eds. *Physicians and Hospitals: The Great Partnership at the Crossroads Based on the Ninth Private Sector Conference, 1985*, p. 95.

[7] David Dranove, *The Economic Evolution of Healthcare. From Marcus Welby to Managed Care*, p. 28.

[8] Ibid., p. 84.

[9] CMS Office of Public Affairs, "Medicare Demonstration Shows Hospital Quality of Care Improves with Payments Tied to Quality."

[10] Ibid.

¹¹ Merrill Goozner, "What Went Wrong?"

¹² News Release, March 30, 2005.

¹³ "HFAP Survey Earns Facility Referral Status: Stays with JCAHO, Now Has Two Certifications."

¹⁴ http://www.skiffmed.com/VITALSIGNS8-5-2004.pdf

¹⁵ http://72.14.203.104/search?q=cache:vxU48opW1WcJ: www.reidhosp.com/news/releases/02032005-okay.html+switched+from+JCAHO+to+HFAP&hl=en&gl=us&ct=clnk&cd=1

¹⁶ "QI Professionals Take Harder Look at Alternatives to JCAHO Accreditation."

¹⁷House Bill #HR4877.

¹⁸ Brauer, p. 121.

¹⁹http://www.jointcommission.org/

²⁰ Brauer, p. 135.

²¹ Joint Commission on Accreditation of Healthcare Organizations. "What is the Joint Commission on Accreditation of Healthcare Organizations?" http://www.jointcommission.org/

²² Ibid.

²³ Gilbert M. Gaul, "Accreditors Blamed for Overlooking Problems," washingtonpost.com, July 25, 2005.

²⁴ Government Accounting Office. Medicare: CMS Needs Additional Authority to Adequately Oversee Patient Safety in Hospitals, July, 2004.

²⁵ http://www.tuvamerica.com/tuvnews/presslist.cfm

²⁶ Lovern

²⁷ Tramontano

²⁸ Lovern